Praise for *Confessions of a Menopausal Woman*

'Love this warm and uplifting read – made me laugh and cry, as well as feel informed and inspired.' Liz Earle

'I love this book. Brilliantly practical, down-to-earth guide about how to not only survive the menopause but to thrive too. Andrea is warm, kind and lovely and it's like sitting down with a good friend who has the best advice.' Suzy Walker, Editor-in-Chief of *Psychologies* magazine

'An inspiration.' *The Lady*

'Invaluable tips and tricks.' *Prima*

'Forget the hours of searching for mixed messages on Dr Google – when it comes to the menopause, this book tells you everything you need to know.' Jane Moore

'This book is so perfect! I have bought it as a gift for many of my friends. They have then, in turn, given it to others. It's been written so honestly and carefully by someone I know and trust. No one else has covered all the areas that Andrea does in her book and covered them so fully and in such an appealing and funny way.' Gaby Roslin

'Andrea has put her heart and soul into this book . . . a bible for all things menopause.' Nadia Sawalha

'I've bought this book for three of my close friends for Christmas. It's such an honest and refreshing read that really helps you to understand the menopause.'
Denise van Outen

'Consider this book a very dear friend as you navigate the menopause . . . It'll hold your hand through the difficult bits and keep you smiling through the rest.' Kaye Adams

'As a young-ish woman experiencing the bewildering, unsettling and sometimes extreme symptoms of peri menopause, all I've wanted is to be able to talk to a girl friend who understands the journey. Someone who's been there, seen it, done that. Someone who can hold your hand, tell you not to worry, and reassure you that you'll come though the other side in time. That is exactly what Andrea has achieved with *Confessions of a Menopausal Woman*. Her warmth and characteristic sensitivity shine through in her honest account of her own suffering – not to be a bleeding heart, but to be a guiding light for other women who are right behind her. Part memoir, part self-help, this book is a must-have-menopause-manual for every girl who wants to feel her best in a time of change.' Anna Richardson

ANDREA MCLEAN
Confessions of a Menopausal Woman

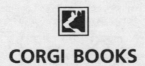

CORGI BOOKS

TRANSWORLD PUBLISHERS
61–63 Uxbridge Road, London W5 5SA
www.penguin.co.uk

Transworld is part of the Penguin Random House group of companies
whose addresses can be found at global.penguinrandomhouse.com

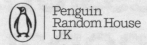

Penguin
Random House
UK

First published in Great Britain in 2018 by Bantam Press
an imprint of Transworld Publishers
Corgi edition published 2019

Copyright © Andrea McLean 2018

Andrea McLean has asserted her right under the Copyright,
Designs and Patents Act 1988 to be identified as the author of this work.

Every effort has been made to obtain the necessary permissions with
reference to copyright material, both illustrative and quoted. We apologize
for any omissions in this respect and will be pleased to make the
appropriate acknowledgements in any future edition.

A CIP catalogue record for this book
is available from the British Library.

ISBN 9780552176477

Typeset in 10.93/14.26pt Minion Pro by Jouve (UK), Milton Keynes.
Printed and bound in Great Britain by Clays Ltd, Elcograf S.p.A.

Penguin Random House is committed to a sustainable
future for our business, our readers and our planet. This book
is made from Forest Stewardship Council® certified paper.

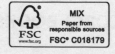

MIX
Paper from
responsible sources
FSC® C018179

1 3 5 7 9 10 8 6 4 2

To menopausal women everywhere.
It's OK. We've got this.

Contents

Introduction

Dear reader,

This is the book I wish I'd had when I started my menopause, and the one I hope will help you through yours . . .

It all began with a thirty-second mention on TV that I was going to be off work for a while, recovering from a hysterectomy. In the space of just two days, *ten thousand* messages came through from viewers, asking to be kept updated; begging for advice, comfort, and for me to share my experience.

I was overwhelmed . . . Over the following weeks, the questions continued to fly in thick and fast, all of them from women desperate for help and support. They wanted to know why I'd needed the hysterectomy, and what the operation had been like, because they were about to have one as well and were scared. Other women were telling me they were in exactly the same situation as me: at home recovering, and feeling overwhelmed by the changes that were happening to their mind and body, the fear of the unknown taking them on a downward spiral of worry and anxiety.

It was clear to me that a huge proportion of the female population in the UK was living in fear and confusion. There was no one for them to talk to about their experience, and no one was helping them.

Take away the word 'menopause' and just look at the symptoms women experience during this time: night sweats, joint and muscle pain, memory loss, depression, fatigue, lethargy, loss of libido. How can *anyone* be expected to carry on a normal life while living in such physical and mental discomfort without support? It's insane when you consider that half the population of the *whole world* will go through this phase of life and be expected to keep a stiff upper lip, not mention anything and simply get on with it. Not talking about things can make us worry that we're the only ones feeling the way we do – and that just makes us feel worse, and even more afraid.

There are pages of information on the internet telling us what to expect physically during the menopause, and what to look out for mentally, but when I started on this journey six years ago there wasn't a book that shared with me how it *felt*, first hand, from someone I knew and trusted. There are some wonderful online forums and sites dedicated to women and their changing needs, but at the time when I personally needed comfort and information, none spoke to me in a voice I liked. Some were frightening and hysterical, if I'm honest, and gave my inner 'what if . . . ?' voice a megaphone to shout at me with, which didn't do much to calm the anxious thoughts zooming around inside my head.

When I went back to work and talked about it on *Loose Women*, the papers picked up on the story and 'Woman Has Menopause' seemed to be, if you'll excuse the pun, pretty hot news. I didn't set out to become the poster girl for all this. It happened by default, because I realized that there wasn't any point pretending that I *hadn't* had a hysterectomy or *wasn't* going through the menopause, and I could see by the response I was getting how much of a relief women were finding it that *someone* was talking about the subject. So, I figured I might as well embrace the conversation that was opening up, and push my experience out there, because some of the information women are being given is scary and headline-grabbing and it really doesn't have to be.

I faced up to the fact that a big part of me was afraid to talk about what I was going through for the same reason that other women in the public eye now confide in me at parties that they too have had hysterectomies, that they too are experiencing 'the change': they don't want anyone to know in case they're seen as being 'old'. These women ask me for advice while swearing me to secrecy at the same time, because they don't want the industry to think that they're now 'past it', and are terrified that they'll be replaced by someone younger and fresher.

Is this because those in positions of power in the entertainment industry truly believe that women over a certain age aren't relevant to viewers at home? Who exactly do they think is 'at home'? While I appreciate that entertainment needs to be aspirational at a certain level – watching other humans do things that we're impressed by (singing, dancing, juggling, answering tricky quiz questions or scaring the life out of politicians, whatever floats your boat . . .) – why does this have a cut-off point for women once they reach 'a certain age'? Why do we have such a culture of youth-centric aspiration?

I've had so many people from all walks of life stop me and thank me for being open about the menopause, for making them feel that they aren't the only ones going through it. Originally, I wasn't going to speak about it publicly because I didn't want to be seen as being old either. I still don't! However, I looked at things again and I shifted my perspective. I saw that this isn't about age – the menopause can happen as early as during your thirties and, my God, if you're old then, what hope does any of us (men included) have!

This whole issue is about women experiencing a life change and being too afraid to ask for help or talk to anyone about it. They want to continue to be seen by the rest of the world – whether that's their workplace or family or friends – as the same vibrant, relevant person they've always been. And it's pretty difficult to feel that way when it seems as if your body is falling apart and your brain has gone for a walk and can't find its way back again.

But you can.

You aren't going to be quite the *same* vibrant, relevant person you were before, but you still have it in you to be absolutely incredible. You'll be different, but different isn't necessarily bad. It's a new stage in life and a new you.

The odd joke about sweating aside, the menopause isn't something we really discuss, and I think that's for a couple of reasons. Firstly, as I've said, it's seen as a sign of impending old age, and no one likes to think of that happening to them before they're ready, right when they're in what feels like the prime of middle age. Secondly, it can make a lot of men feel uncomfortable, so we end up keeping quiet and soldiering on.

The menopause doesn't always mean advancing years – in any case, fifty (the average age for a woman to reach the menopause) isn't old. And in the case of men's hang-ups, well, it doesn't have to be this way, and I think things can change. They don't have to be squeamish about what's going on with women's bodies – it all comes down to education and being armed with the right information. And that's where you and I come in.

Talking about stuff is what women do best. We share and offload, we laugh and we bond over the ridiculous and incredible things our bodies go through, and hearing other people's experiences is what makes our own so much more bearable – we are not alone! We shouldn't keep this stuff to ourselves.

That's why I wanted to share my story, and the stories of those women who got in touch with me: to show you that life after a hysterectomy, and after the menopause, isn't quite the same. It can be scary, horrible, irritating and draining . . . but it can also be transformative and liberating, if you change how you look at it and get the help you need.

It's all about experience and perspective – and as a woman who has chosen to make her living out of sharing experiences and giving a different perspective, it made total sense to me to write this book . . . once I'd got my head around the fact that I would have to be really, *really* open about myself.

This book is a chat, a conversation that will move from humour to sadness and back again, with all the information I've gathered through experience and research as its backbone, plus expert advice from a medical professional who is as convinced as I am that women need to be given genuinely helpful information so they can make informed decisions about their health and well-being. Don't we all want to have a friend who can talk us through stuff and tell us it's going to be all right? And don't you always trust the words of a friend who has been through it herself, rather than something written by a faceless 'expert' you've come across online? I know I do.

I'm a big sister, a daughter, a mother and a friend. I'm all of those things to people I love, and I hope I can be that to you, too. I've been on the hormone rollercoaster (some days I'm still on it!) and I'm here to tell you that some bits will turn you upside down, and some twists and turns you won't see coming, but it will all be fine in the end. I hope I can help you enjoy the ride . . .

With love,

Andrea x

1

What Is the Menopause?

So, what is the menopause? Ask a hundred people and you'll get a hundred different answers to that one! So I asked 200,000 people, through the magic of social media, by putting the following question to my Facebook and Twitter followers: 'What does the word "menopause" mean to you?' The response I got was a tsunami of symptoms and feelings, from women who felt helpless, anxious and lost.

Here are a few of them. I've kept them anonymous as, understandably, not all women want to let the world know what they're going through.

'It means I'm not who I used to be. Flushes, night sweats, mood swings. For me the worst has been the impact on my memory and concentration, and the impact on my career.'

'Lack of understanding. Lack of consideration to symptoms. Many women just have to carry on as normal, even though their body and mind are doing strange things.'

'I cried because I realized, "That's it for me, children are grown and gone", and the feeling of being old for the first time in my life. Then came the terrible, terrible hot sweats . . .'

'Don't feel like me any more. Fatigue, muscle and joint aches, so bloated, low mood, forgetful, emotional.'

They're just a tiny fraction of the responses I got, and I'll sprinkle more of them throughout this book, and try to reference as many of them as I can.

After I'd consulted the Twittersphere, I then did what anyone else does when they want to know the answer to something: I typed 'What is the menopause?' into Google. In 0.61 seconds it offered me 24.3 million results and I didn't read one that made me feel any better.

Technically speaking, according to NHS Choices, 'The menopause is when a woman stops having periods and is no longer able to get pregnant naturally . . . [It's] a natural part of ageing that usually occurs between forty-five and fifty-five years of age, as a woman's oestrogen levels decline. In the UK, the average age for a woman to reach the menopause is fifty-one.'

Mean anything to you? No, me either. It's about as useful as reading a biology textbook at school to understand why you feel wretched once a month. The medical definition gives you the theory, but what we really want to know is what the reality is like. When I had a coil for seven years, I didn't have periods with it, so how was I to know whether they had actually stopped or not? Surely there's more to a menopause diagnosis than the absence of a monthly cycle?

Given that our periods stop because of declining oestrogen levels, one of the first things you need to know is what oestrogen is. In the simplest terms, it's a sex hormone produced by women, which is responsible for the developmental changes the female body undergoes during puberty.

As well as regulating our menstrual cycle, it also affects how our skin looks and how strong our bones are, amongst other things.

When you dig a bit deeper, you discover that the build-up to the *actual* menopause can take years. There's a period of time before it really kicks in, when the symptoms start to build. The BUPA website states:

The menopause is a natural change in a woman's life; it happens when your ovaries stop producing eggs. Your ovaries also make the hormone oestrogen (a chemical substance). So when they stop working, there's a drop in your blood level of this hormone. This change disrupts your periods and causes the symptoms associated with the menopause.

The menopause usually happens gradually. For a few years before the menopause, your periods may become irregular, happening more or less often than they used to. You may also have slightly heavier periods. This stage is called the perimenopause and can last for about four years. You can still become pregnant while going through the perimenopause, so you need to keep using contraception if you don't want to get pregnant. Doctors usually recommend stopping contraception at fifty-five, because most women are in the menopause by this age.

You're said to have reached the menopause if you haven't had a period for at least a year. When the menopause happens before the age of forty, it's considered to be premature (early) menopause. An early menopause can happen naturally because your ovaries stop working. But it can also happen if you've had one or both of your ovaries removed as part of a hysterectomy (an operation to remove your womb).*

Like anything, each one of us will experience the build-up to the menopause in our own unique way. While there will be some uniting factors (getting hot, sweaty, anxious and grumpy seem to be the main ones), there's a whole host of symptoms and experiences that come under the umbrella term of 'menopause'.

I hope you're beginning to get the picture of what it's all about, but if you're still none the wiser then take a look at this list. There are apparently thirty-four signs of being menopausal – either peri-, which is the build-up, or full-blown. They are:

Allergies Any you have seem stronger than usual.

Anxiety and stress

Bladder incontinence

Bleeding gums

Bloating

Breast tenderness

Brittle nails

Body odour changes Sweating more, and a change in your 'normal smell'.

Burning tongue or dry mouth

Depression

Difficulty concentrating

Dizziness

Electric shocks Tingling sensation under the skin – often across the head, but also in the back.

Gastrointestinal problems Gas, cramping and nausea.

Hot flushes

Hair changes Increase in facial hair, but thinning hair elsewhere.

Headaches Especially at the start of the menopause.

Irregular menstrual cycle

* www.bupa.co.uk/health-information/directory/m/menopause

Irregular, pounding heartbeat
Irritability
Itchy skin
Joint pain
Loss of libido
Memory lapses
Mood swings
Muscle tension
Night sweats
Osteoporosis A condition that weakens the bones.
Overwhelming fatigue
Panic attacks
Sleep disorders
Tingling extremities
Vaginal dryness
Weight gain

How joyful does all that sound?! Does reading the list and ticking the symptoms off one by one make you feel like curling into a ball and giving up, because there it is in black and white? Is there no denying it any longer – the proof right in front of your eyes? Are you officially menopausal?

Or is this your ta-da moment? A realization that you're *not* going mad, that there *is* a reason behind the feelings and physical sensations you're experiencing. Now you know for sure, reading on in this book might be your first step towards doing something about it, and making yourself feel better, both mentally and physically.

I have pretty much all those symptoms, and for a while I didn't know if discovering they're all related to the menopause made me feel better or worse. Now I've got my head around it, I know I feel better because – well, for one thing, I can show this list to my other half and explain that it's not my fault I'm forgetful, distracted, irritable, fat, sweaty, smelly, panicky, hairy – and hairless. In fact, I may even print it off and stick it to the fridge . . .

This is where I think talking about our experiences is so important. Knowing what is happening to us from a biological point of view is all well and good – and really helpful resources such as the NHS or BUPA websites can give us that core information – but how are you left *feeling* on a day-to-day basis? And then what can you do about it? I don't want to just roll over and accept that this is the 'new me' any more than I want to accept that my hair is actually grey. Sod that! I suspect many of you feel the same.

Back in the day . . .

My mum was forty when she started her journey through the menopause. I can remember her becoming increasingly short-tempered with me and my sister, culminating in some sharp words in the car one day. Dad pulled over and stopped, as Mum glared out the window, looking thunderous.

'Girls,' he said, as he turned to face us in the back seat, 'your mum is going through "the change" and we all need to be a bit more patient with her. OK? That means no winding each other up, and be nice, all right?'

We nodded, and nothing more was said. Ever. I had no idea what this 'change' was, but it didn't seem great. Mum eventually calmed down (thanks to HRT, I found out later), and family life returned to normal.

I asked my mum recently about her memories of that time. She told me she mainly remembers crying more (my mum is not a crier) and just not feeling like herself. When she went to see her (male) GP, he told her it was just her age and that was that. There was nothing to be done. Not long after that, we moved away from the area, so she had to change surgeries, and her new (female) doctor immediately told her she needed HRT. Within weeks she started to feel better, and she kept taking the treatment for the next fifteen years. She also told me she didn't know what the menopause was when *her* mum went through it, also at the age of forty. She can't recall my grandmother ever mentioning it until years after she'd come out the other side.

So, from the 1960s when my granny went through her menopause, to the eighties when my mum started hers, right up to the present day, very little appears to have changed. It's a great shame for us all that society doesn't seem to have moved much further forward in its attitudes since my grandmother's generation. In our supposedly enlightened times, when we're apparently free to be who we wanna be and do what we wanna do, we *still* don't talk about it. Those of us old enough to remember the Primal Scream song 'Loaded' (and the sample of Peter Fonda's infamous quote from the film *The Wild Angels*), will remember shaking our sweaty heads to it in nightclubs in the 1990s. Or maybe you've just heard it on the radio. Either way, the words have always stayed with me.

This 'can-do' attitude only seems to apply if you're young and restless, shaking things up a little; not if you're middle-aged. And certainly not if you're a middle-aged woman. How ridiculous. How can such a huge proportion of the population simply not count, just because they've reached the second (amazing) phase of their adult lives and have half a lifetime of experience, knowledge and expertise to offer?

It seems to have become so ingrained in us as a society to think of women as quietly acquiescing – firstly to our parents, then to our partners and bosses, and eventually to our children's needs – that the thought of us reaching a point in our lives where we feel strong and capable enough to say 'no' goes against the grain. By this I mean some women – and in particular women now in middle age – have been raised to keep quiet about what we want, need or feel, because we've been conditioned to believe the wants, needs or feelings of others are more important than ours. In essence, it means when we're asked if we're OK, we say, 'Yes I'm fine,' rather than 'No, I'm struggling . . .' Of course this isn't the norm for everyone, but for my grandmother and mother's generations, and yes, also in some cases for ours, there's certainly a ring of truth to it.

Think about it. We tell our daughters that they can do anything that boys can do. We encourage them to try hard at school, achieve academically and get a good job, then the minute they get to their twenties or thirties the world pressures them into finding a man, settling down and having children – essentially putting their dreams and abilities second. Of course, a lot of this is to do with social conditioning; how we've been raised by our parents, how we've observed our mother behaving, and whether we've decided subconsciously to follow her example or do the exact opposite.

Even now, with the average age of first-time mums being over thirty, the press poke and speculate wildly over every fresh-faced starlet's thoughts on getting engaged and settling down, asking if she yearns for the pitter-patter of tiny feet, all within hours of her snogging someone on reality TV. We're so used to seeing it and reading about it, that it doesn't even register as being an odd way to look at things. And that's the media's attitude towards today's young women, in 2018. By the time we enter our middle years, filled with all the knowledge life has afforded us, society has deemed us too old to be relevant.

So far so apparently normal, but imagine if men were subjected to those same kinds of skewed attitudes and pressures. Would society consider a middle-aged man to be 'past it' once he'd successfully raised a family and negotiated a career ladder against a ticking clock and ingrained prejudice against his thinning hair and thickening middle? A man's greying hair and laughter lines show how distinguished he is, his advancing years are testament to his knowledge and wisdom – he's far from past it, he's just getting into his stride!

So why have we accepted and, through the generations, perpetuated the notion that the way middle-aged women are viewed by society is the norm? Is it because rebellion is the prerogative of the young? As someone who has been a 'good girl' her whole life, raised to please and turn the other cheek, I am as surprised as anyone at how angry this expected acquiescence over something that is such a fundamental part of being a woman has made me. The menopause has fired me up, in *every* way.

The menopause and me

The word 'menopause' first crept into my vocabulary when I was forty-two. I'd heard about it, obviously, but directly related to me? No. I'd been having night sweats since my late thirties; waking up with saturated sheets, my pyjamas wringing wet. I was told it was my hormones playing up – whatever that means – and that they'd soon calm down. They didn't. I fell pregnant instead! I later learned that a last 'rush' of fertility hormones is fairly common in women during the perimenopause.

My body went haywire for a while after that. Things settled down again after the birth of my lovely daughter, but then I suffered from postnatal depression and acute stress and anxiety as my marriage ended. During that time, it was pretty hard to separate out high emotion and 'normal' stress – which we all experience; it's when you know that you're going to come out the other side – from symptoms linked to the menopause. But I knew I wasn't feeling right.

A few years previously, around the time of my fortieth birthday and when my night sweats and non-existent libido had made it clear that something was definitely not right, I'd been recommended a gynaecologist in London by the name of Professor John Studd. He's been a champion of women's health for his whole career, and is evangelical in his drive for women to be listened to and given the care and support they need when it comes to managing PMS and the menopause.

When I went to see him, Professor Studd did some blood and bone-density tests, and revealed that I was indeed peri-menopausal. He prescribed some oestrogen gel, which I took for a time and my symptoms eased. Then, to be honest, any thoughts about potential menopausal symptoms were put to one side as life got in the way. It's pretty hard to nail down the precise cause of your anxiety, depression, stress, upset, rage and lack of libido when your marriage is ending!

I had no interest in starting a relationship with anyone, so being on my own meant I didn't have much of a barometer as to how my libido was faring anyway. However, the sweats came back and I was definitely feeling worse than before. I needed to get things sorted. A year or so later, a chance encounter with the wonderful Dr Tina Peers changed everything and I finally got to the heart of it all.

How do you know you're menopausal?

I was sent to Dr Peers because when the time came to replace my Mirena coil, my GP couldn't remove it. It was 'stuck'. After a lot of uncomfortable tugging and rummaging around, my GP eventually sent me to a day hospital to see Dr Peers, as she's an expert in all things down below. And that turn of fate changed my life!

Dr Peers is a Consultant in Contraception and Reproductive Health, with a special interest in menopause management. She's passionate about helping women to feel as well as they possibly can and finding the best way to treat them. Once she'd replaced my coil and examined me, we sat and talked about how I was doing. What a relief! She was around the same age as me, sympathetic, and understood right away what I meant when I described my night sweats, anxiety, lack of concentration and the overall feeling that I wasn't 'me' any more.

I gave her the blood test results from when I'd seen Professor Studd a few years previously, and told her that the oestrogen gel had made a big difference to me. Even though I was still technically young to be starting the menopause, it wasn't an outrageous thought either. My mum had been forty when she started hers; I was now forty-three. So, Dr Peers prescribed me the same Sandrena gel that Professor Studd had; an HRT (hormone replacement therapy) gel, where oestrogen is the main hormone being replaced – you just rub it into your skin once a day and it gets absorbed – and recommended that I speak to my GP about getting a repeat prescription.

My original appointments with Dr Peers had been on the NHS, who then promptly stopped funding treatment for women like me who were 'not quite there yet'. Probably due to funding issues, I and other perimenopausal women now had to fall off the menopausal cliff and wait until we were in free-fall in order to qualify for treatment. When I saw my GP for a repeat prescription, Dr Peers's notes to him showed that I was perimenopausal rather than in the full throes.

However, never one to take no for an answer, I pointed out to him that the blood tests had been taken a few years previously, and my symptoms were now worse than ever. Reluctantly, this male doctor prescribed me the same Sandrena oestrogen gel that Dr Peers had put me on. I started off using one sachet a day, and was told to increase the dosage to what felt right for me. That's the thing: there is no standard prescription for hormonal irregularities. So much of it comes down to not feeling 'right', and only we know what feels right for us. It took time, and some adjusting of the dosage, but I got there eventually. The medication attacked the symptoms but left me still feeling like myself.

And what I felt was much, much better! Starting HRT was as life-changing at forty-three as going on the pill had been at nineteen: the sweats stopped, I gradually became more balanced, my moods evened out and lifted, and my anxiety returned to its normal level. Normal for me, that is – it was still there but I could function. I felt like I was sailing on calm waters again. My hair was still thinning and there were terrible patches where, in the wrong light, I could see my scalp but, hey, if that was the worst thing, I could put up with it. That's what make-up and hair extensions are for anyway!

The perimenopause

The perimenopause seems to me to be treated like a bit of a 'meh' thing; it's just something that women are expected to put up with while waiting for the *real* menopause to kick in, at which point they can properly ask for help. But here's the thing: the perimenopause can last for over a *decade*! Who the hell wants to feel terrible for a huge chunk of their life, waiting until things get bad enough for a doctor to decide they're ready for medication to make them feel better? I truly don't understand the logic of that.

In a way, the perimenopause can be even worse than the menopause itself, because it's not seen as a big enough thing to receive treatment for, but in the meantime you're left feeling wretched. Antidepressants get handed out like Smarties but actually, some replacement hormones would help, because it's your hormones that are out of whack. The difficulty is, I suppose, understanding your symptoms well enough to know if what you're feeling is actually the start of the menopause or something else entirely.

To help with my research for this book, I spoke to Dr Peers and asked her a few questions. Look out for her input at the end of each chapter and in the Appendix on page 231–42, which ensures that as well as getting a friendly take on the menopause, you're also getting some vital medical information.

Apparently, the typical age of a woman who comes to see Dr Peers is late forties to early fifties. These patients' symptoms are affecting their quality of life and starting to interfere with their ability to function well. In other words, they've put up with them until they've become unbearable because, let's face it, women can put up with an awful lot before we buckle!

In terms of their physical symptoms, these women are experiencing the exact same things as the women who got in touch with me after my hysterectomy: hot flushes, night sweats, poor-quality sleep, palpitations, aching joints and muscles. Mentally, the women mention irritability, tearfulness, forgetfulness, memory loss and poor concentration. All these things look pretty awful when you see them together on the page in black and white. The thing is, you don't have to put up with them.

To HRT or not to HRT?
That is the burning question . . .

I asked Dr Peers about HRT, and the drug she'd prescribed me – can it really help women with both their physical and mental symptoms? Her answer was an unequivocal yes. According to her, the oestrogen absorbed through the skin stimulates our oestrogen receptors to 'switch on' various types of cells again – ones that produce collagen or bone, for example. The result of their activity then leads to a reduction in various symptoms.

The problem with HRT is the bad press it's received over the years, with headlines linking it to an increase in breast cancer being the most worrying. Surely it's understandable that women are worried about using it, and that GPs are reluctant to prescribe it?

Dr Peers told me that in the eighties and nineties, around the time she first qualified as a doctor, women were happily taking HRT for many years. As a GP, she had many patients who stayed on HRT for fifteen to twenty years. The Women's Health Initiative study in 2002 changed this. 'It overstated risks,' she explained. 'Many of which were not statistically significant and did not take account of confounding factors, in a very poorly designed study.'

So, if that's the case, and the opinion of a respected women's health professional, how do you change the perception of HRT and reassure women that it *is* safe to use? Dr Peers's response to this question was simple, and can be summed up in one word: education. Whether that's through correct and

accurate information on the internet, leaflets in doctors' surgeries, or ensuring GPs' and nurses' knowledge is up to date.

And if women would still prefer *not* to use HRT? Then
diet, exercise, food and therapy are all recommended, plus
cognitive behavioural therapy (CBT), reducing alcohol intake
and losing weight. These are all treatments and solutions that
I'll be looking into in much more detail, later on in this book.

A *change gonna come*

From the moment we get our first period, all the way through
to our last, we're conditioned not to talk about them – even
woman to woman, never mind around men. There's a secrecy
surrounding the menstrual cycle, a gentle pretence that maybe
it's not really happening and, if it is, it's all absolutely fine, even
when it isn't.

Then we get to the other end of the spectrum. Sweating and
'being menopausal' in the workplace is too much for everyone
to handle, which is incredibly isolating. Why can't we talk about
it? Is it because it involves blood? Is it because it's icky and yuk,
and not pleasant, and men find it scary, and, let's be honest,
women *can* get a bit strange at certain times of the month?

I think we need to take responsibility for the fact that we're
driven by hormones. By that I mean we are of course aware of
it – it's biology after all – but do we properly acknowledge it? Do
we look it in the eye and own up to our thoughts and actions
being different at certain moments in the month compared to
others? We know that many men see themselves as consistent
creatures and see women as inconsistent. Perhaps we need to
admit that, to a point, at times, they might be right? Our bodies
are complicated. Something that irritates you one day will slide

over you the next. That's a fact. That really happens. So rather than pretending it doesn't, or getting defensive if it's alluded to, surely it's better to acknowledge it and work with it?

I appreciate that some people will object to the idea that they're ruled by their hormones. However, I think that's perhaps because women have been made to feel that it's a bad thing, when it's just the way it is. It's a natural part of human biology and happens to us all to a lesser or greater extent – men included. Nevertheless, somewhere along the path of our evolution into apparently sophisticated beings, hormonal behaviour has become something to be suppressed or hidden, particularly when it pertains to women. Just look at how it's spoken about, in that sarcastic 'Ooh, is it that time of the month, love?' kind of way.

Those hormonal emotions – anger, frustration, anxiety, fear, depression – tend to be viewed negatively. Society openly denigrates women for displaying them, and regards us as the 'weaker sex' for doing so. But just looking at this logically, it's not only half the species that experiences these feelings. We all do – both men and women. Men themselves are made to feel weak and unmanly for showing anxiety, fear and depression, and society's reaction is one of the key contributing factors of male suicide in the UK today. We're made to feel that any deviation from the so-called and socially accepted norm is unacceptable. Which is heartbreaking for all of us.

All the important conversations that are happening about what we should and shouldn't accept in the workplace, particularly when it comes to inappropriate and sexist behaviour, are opening doors to deeper discussions about the reality of what it means to be a woman. Damn right the time has come for women to stand up and say 'time's up' for being treated as inconsequential bit-part players. I stand shoulder to shoulder with my fellow women on this – sexism, misogyny and bigotry are appalling, infuriating and make me want to punch walls in frustration. This is the perfect moment for women's needs to be owned and addressed, rather than hidden away. We're living at a time when we have never been in a more powerful position to stand up against inequality and demand equal pay, rights and standards. Which is fantastic. Although we're different, that doesn't mean we're not equal, which is why it makes me so angry that the way women are treated during the menopause has been unacknowledged for so long.

The menopause is an important marker of change for a woman, and comes at a point in most women's lives when we're just becoming sure of ourselves in terms of what we want, and what we don't. It's a stage of life when we're starting to be less fussed about what others think of us, and have enough life experience to care less about whether we're doing what other people think we should.

However, rather than this confidence being seen as a gift, society knocks us back with the very thing we should be waving in the air – our age, experience and ability to cope with what Mother Nature has given us so bloody brilliantly. And yes, I'm talking about almost a lifetime of monthly periods here . . . We are the stronger sex, there's no doubt about that in my mind. By 'stronger', I mean that we are born with the same mental capabilities as the male of the species but also with the physical ability to bear children, and therefore keep the human race on this planet.

This means the female body is made differently: it has to be able to change and fluctuate physically and mentally as it prepares for the moment it might be called upon to reproduce.

Our bodies are constantly on call, then on high alert once a month, ready for action. It's no wonder we feel a bit up and down! And yet, throughout all these physical changes, part of our brain is still carrying on as usual as we go to work, make decisions, deal with family, and manage all the other thousands of daily tasks we do without even noticing. Forget being *embarrassed* about the physical fluctuations that our bodies and mind cope with, we should be *proud*!

Now, I'm a big believer in balance in all things. Just like I don't go to the gym every day, and wouldn't dream of turning down a glass of plonk because water is so much better for me, I don't think we need to go from hiding our feminine experience to waving it under everyone's nose all the time. I am strong on this point – not everyone wants or needs to know our business. I feel the same way about people who have a cold, or a sore toe, or feel the need to shove their political beliefs down everyone's throat – I don't need to hear every last detail of their illness or whether they voted Leave or Remain, and nor do I want to.

What I *do* think needs to change is the unspoken acceptance that one-third of a woman's life is irrelevant or embarrassing. This is born of ignorance on so many sides: in the medical world, where some doctors try to sweep the menopause under the carpet – and they need to be educated; in the professional world, where older women are eased out of jobs; and in our personal lives too, where some women entering their middle years are traded in for younger, firmer, perhaps more compliant models. With knowledge comes power, and one of the best ways to gain that knowledge is through shared experience.

I totally understand why some women choose not to discuss the menopause, or admit to going through it, because of the connotations of ageing and becoming an old lady who is a figure of fun and derision rather than a capable female of the species. With respect and support from our partners in love, friends in life and colleagues at work, I'm hopeful that 'the change' can become something to be embraced as a new chapter rather than being seen as the beginning of the end.

I think one of the ways we can begin to instigate a change in attitudes is for us mums to educate our sons about what women are really all about. I talk to my teenage son about how his body and mindset alter because of hormonal changes, and how women go through the same thing – he needs to know that. It's common sense and basic biology to explain to them what's going on – not just in your teens, but all the way through your life.

If the next generation of educated boys grow up to become enlightened men, I'm hopeful that my daughter, when her time comes, won't have to fear mentioning 'the change' in case she's thought of as old and past it by her peers. Hopefully by then, there will be more people in general, both male *and* female, who will see it for what it is: a normal part of life. It's the menopause.

Dr Peers Says . . .

THE CASE FOR HRT

Hormone replacement therapy does exactly as its name suggests: it replaces the hormone that your body stops producing when you go through the menopause – oestrogen. It can be taken as tablets, as a gel rubbed into your skin, as a long-lasting implant, or – for local oestrogen to improve the vaginal, vulval and bladder health – as a vaginal pessary or cream.

HRT is the most effective way of relieving menopausal symptoms and it also reduces the risk of osteoporosis.[1]

The Women's Health Initiative study (WHI) in 2002 dramatically changed attitudes towards HRT. 'The study raised concerns about safety and caused panic amongst the women taking HRT and confusion for the doctors prescribing it. However, the WHI study had overstated the risks – many were not statistically significant, neither did they allow for confounding factors such as age and the time women started to take HRT. Further analysis of the study a few years later highlighted these issues but the damage had already been done. As a result, many women have missed out on treatment of their menopausal symptoms.'[2]

[1] Source: Women's Health Concern. HRT. www.womens-health-concern.org/help-and-advice/factsheets/hrt/

[2] Source: Women's Health Concern. HRT – Understanding benefits and risks. www.womens-health-concern.org/help-and-advice/factsheets/hrt-know-benefits-risks/

2

Whose Body Is This Anyway?

....

'An absolute nightmare. Hot sweats, memory loss, lack of sleep. There seems to be no end. I wouldn't wish it on my worst enemy.'

'Dreading a sneeze, bracing myself with crossed legs, weak bladder. Leg in, leg out of the bed. Sweaty hair, mood swings, sweet cravings, headaches, bloating and weight gain. What a joy . . . And how long does it last? No one knows . . .'

'To me, menopause is a timely reminder to listen to your body and make some changes to ensure you stay healthy and strong through your menopause years and beyond. One hundred per cent of women will go through menopause and we shouldn't feel embarrassed or ashamed to talk about it.'
The Menopause Coach

....

Glorious hormones

Ah, the menopause. 'The change'. Women's troubles. All brought to you and me in glorious Technicolor by those powerful little messenger molecules we call hormones. Before I walk you through my 'change', to see how it compares to yours, I'd like to take you back a bit – to the start, if you like – to where my journey with hormones began and, for the first time but not the last, my body felt as though it had a mind of its own . . .

As a teenager, hormones brought with them delightful acne, which spread across my face, chest and back in angry red pustules that were every bit as gruesome as they sound. My mum has only recently admitted to me that she wishes she'd kept me off school some days to let particularly angry spots on my face die down; if only so that I could see again out of the eye that had been forced shut by the size of the spot by my eye socket. Yes, it really was that bad.

I tried every cream and lotion the eighties had to offer, and spent my school days with my face painted Oompa-Loompa orange. I don't think that was technically what that particular shade of Body Shop foundation was called, but it was certainly that hue. I tried anything to hide the angry bumps – creams, powders and blushes – but, as we all know, they don't really work. I was put on powerful prescription pills for acne that dried my skin and made it sore and red, but didn't do much for the spots themselves. I tried nail-polish remover, dabbed on with a cotton bud, to dry them out. Blobs of toothpaste. Still they bubbled to the surface. Between my lumpen face and the home haircut and perm from my mum, from the neck up the eighties were a beauty disaster for me.

Somehow I got myself a boyfriend. I can only assume my twinkling personality made up for what I looked like because, just before my nineteenth birthday, I decided to move my relationship with him to the next level. The time felt right, so I took myself to the doctor and was given a prescription for the pill. I went on Marvelon, an oral contraceptive that, unbeknown to me, was also being used to treat women with acne.

The results were incredible. To say it was life-changing isn't an exaggeration. For someone who'd been known as 'spotty' all through secondary school to finally have clear skin was incredible! My spots disappeared within a few months, and other than a few bumps that appeared once a month – and the normal sort of pimples that appeared for no good reason – my skin looked like everyone else's. I didn't experience any side effects being on the pill – I felt exactly the same, just spot- and pregnancy-free!

Discovering endometriosis

Fast-forward ten years and at twenty-eight, after experiencing many years of pain down below, I realized that what I was feeling wasn't the same as other women's menstrual cramps. The pain wasn't just during my 'time of the month', it was there all the time. After sex and during my period it was an intense stabbing that took my breath away, and the rest of the time it was a dull, throbbing ache that never really went away.

I went to my GP and got a referral to a gynaecologist, who sent me for a laparoscopy to see what was going on. The results were conclusive: I had endometriosis, a condition where the kind of tissue that normally lines your uterus grows in places outside of it too. My left fallopian tube was riddled with it, and I also had cysts on my ovaries.

As I sat in front of my gynaecologist, a middle-aged man wearing an ill-judged bow tie, he informed me that it would 'take a miracle' for me to get pregnant. He said it quite casually, as though he was letting me know I was wearing an eyeshadow that didn't quite suit me. I asked if there was anything

I could do to help me conceive, and he said I would need fertility treatment. However, I'd need to try to conceive naturally for at least a year in order to qualify for it on the NHS.

This news hit me like a truck. All my young adult years had been spent trying not to get pregnant, and now, in an instant – in that split second – *nothing* would be the same again. I gathered my things and walked out of the hospital doors into a world that, to me, had forever changed. Every other person seemed to be pushing a pram, holding a toddler's hand, or absent-mindedly stroking a swollen, baby-filled belly. It's a difficult one to put into words if you've never experienced it, but the feeling of loss and grief for something I might never be able to have, that I'd taken for granted would happen 'someday', was overwhelming. I made my way home, sat at the kitchen table and cried.

When my boyfriend got home from work, he found a red-eyed but determined wreck. I wanted to have a baby. Not now, not immediately. But at some point. And I knew I wanted to have one with him. I loved him; we'd been together since we were seventeen. We'd bought a flat together, and the assumption was (at least in my mind) that we would carry on being a couple. But finding out that it could take years (if it happened at all) to get pregnant meant that I had to put some serious thought into where our relationship was going.

I did the maths . . . I'd always thought I'd be married and settled down before having children, and if it was going to take years for that to happen, it meant we were going to have to talk about the getting married bit sooner rather than later. He paced the kitchen as I cried and told him what the doctor had said, and my thoughts on what we should do.

His response wasn't the one I was expecting. He didn't rush over, gather me into his arms and drop down on one knee . . .

he looked horrified. This wasn't in his plans *at all*. He didn't want to get married because he still wasn't sure about us, and he wasn't ready to settle down. Ever.

If me announcing that, after eleven years together, I wanted us to move to the next stage of our relationship was a shock to him, him telling me that he *wasn't sure about us* was a massive shock to me. I fell apart. In the end we had a huge row and I told him that if he didn't know after all this time whether he wanted to be with me or not, then he'd better figure it out pretty damn soon, because I wasn't going to waste my time hanging round while he made his mind up. I told him he had six months to decide, and if he didn't think he could commit to me, then we would be going our separate ways.

It was a tense time, as you can imagine. So, a few months later, on my twenty-ninth birthday, when he *did* drop to one knee and propose, I was over the moon. He *did* want me!

No-baby blues – then and now

Anyone who has felt the overwhelming urge to have a baby will understand what it means to have your body and mind ruled by hormones. Obviously the first time that hormones affect a female's thoughts and behaviour comes with the arrival of a girl's first period. That's the moment when *everything* changes. However, the first time a woman really starts to think about having her own babies – rather than seeing having children as something that occurs in other people's lives, or which may or may not happen in her own at some unspecified point in the future – is when a strong hormonal drive comes to the fore. When that surge happens, the tick-tock of that biological clock is deafening.

It's at this point that it becomes clear that, no matter what

31

ideas we have about how evolved we are as a sex, a species or a society, the female is driven to procreate – the human race is depending on it! I completely acknowledge that not every woman experiences this – we are all unique beings after all, whose life experiences are as individual as we are. But for many, this drive is a strong and compelling force of nature.

The second time it rears its head with such intensity is when it becomes apparent that our bodies are coming to the end of their ability to reproduce; when the hormones that have prepared our bodies for pregnancy every month since the transition from girl to woman start to recede. It's a big moment – it's not called 'the change' for nothing.

In my case, a few years after my endometriosis diagnosis and emotional meltdown, I was married and ready to start trying for a baby. I came off the pill and started monitoring my periods. Once I was having them naturally for the first time in years, I discovered that, actually, I rarely had them. They were all over the place, completely sporadic. Eighteen months later, unsurprisingly, I still hadn't conceived. Interestingly, it didn't occur to me to request treatment for my endometriosis, which might have helped matters (as well as the pain I was in constantly). I focused purely on fertility treatment. I just wanted a baby.

I returned to my bow-tied consultant and he put me on Clomid (clomiphene), a fertility drug which causes the release of hormones that stimulate the monthly release of an egg from one of the ovaries. It's a short-term treatment for women who are either not ovulating regularly or who aren't ovulating at all. The best way to describe Clomid is that it makes your body feel like it's in a rush. I could literally feel the hormones and blood whooshing around my body, and my heart pumping in my chest as it got to work on making those eggs pop.

It was like a mini-menopause and I was all over the place – happy one minute, down the next; full of energy, then exhausted. My hormones were having a field day. Up, down, up, down, for months and months on end. I kept a stiff-ish upper lip throughout it all, and tried to keep my hormonal explosions under wraps, like a superhero does when they throw themselves over a bomb. Nothing to see here . . . Nothing to see . . .

Every six weeks or so I'd go back to the consultant and we'd talk through dosages, my periods (which were now happening fairly regularly) and my lack of pregnancy. I'm making this sound all very matter-of-fact, though it was anything but. It put a huge strain on me and my husband as a couple, because sex had gone from being something that happened when the moment took us, to something that we had to do when the time was right. You probably know the feeling.

This was years before fertility-tracking apps and things like that, so all I had were symbols in my diary to mark when I was due to start my period, when I actually started and, crucially, when I was at my most fertile. This window usually came at the most awkward time – when we were like ships in the night with work, me getting up at 3.30 a.m. to head into *GMTV*, and him working normal, long hours during the day.

A year passed, and nothing.

Just when I was about to take things up a notch with the fertility treatment, I went to stay with my sister. Our whole family was there, helping her prepare for her wedding. My dad was doing most of the driving as we ran errands, and I was sitting in the back feeling carsick (like I always do when he drives), when a thought crossed my mind. I'd been feeling a little 'off' and my boobs hurt, but I'd had fertility drugs racing round my body for so long that I was used to feeling out of sorts.

When we got to the town centre, we split up and I headed for Boots to buy a pregnancy test. The nearest loos were in Debenhams so it was there, by myself, that I first saw the positive result appear on the stick. I was so overwhelmed I didn't know whether to laugh or cry. I went straight back to Boots and bought two more tests, just in case. Then I met up with the rest of my family and didn't say a word – I didn't want to take the spotlight away from my sister; this was her moment not mine. But it had happened. I was pregnant!

After a few early hiccups, the pregnancy went well. I was rushed in to see my consultant at one point early on, as I was in so much pain they thought the pregnancy might be ectopic. However, after examining me, and after an ultrasound scan showed the baby was where it should be, the consultant advised me that it was probably hormones rushing to the area where the adhesions resulting from my endometriosis were that was causing the pain. I took paracetamol and hoped for the best.

And the best thing did happen: my beautiful baby boy was born. The fact that I was able to become a mother was something I was happily grateful for at the time, but the full enormity of the privilege of being able to have children only really hit home years later as I recovered from my hysterectomy. As a result of the surgery I had no womb, no ovaries, and my body was tumbling headlong into menopause. There were no specialists I could see to change the fact that having any more children was officially no longer an option.

Many women will recognize this feeling once their body has entered its full menopausal stage; whether through a medically induced menopause, as happens following a hysterectomy, or naturally. The pain is real and deep, and I'm grateful and thankful that I was able to conceive before that chance was fully taken away from me.

Hormones and postnatal depression

Five years after my son was born, I became pregnant again. This time I didn't need any fertility treatment at all, which was such a shock but incredible. I hadn't even considered that I'd be able to have any children without it. I did, though, and I'm blessed to have had two pregnancies and two healthy children. To be honest, I didn't want to push my luck after that, and I always felt that I'd had my share. A boy and a girl. Who could ask for more?

Managing my hormones following the birth of my daughter became a different issue. I developed postnatal depression and if I'm honest, looking back on it now, I think there were a number of factors at play, not just my hormones, though they certainly played a huge part. The postnatal hormonal dip sent me crashing downwards, and everything I'd tried to cope with just couldn't be squashed down any more. It was a horrible experience, but if there was one thing to be glad about during that time, it was that it didn't affect my love for my baby. I adored her; it was *me* I didn't like.

I kept quiet about my feelings of hopelessness and futility for years, and tried to deal with it myself. I thought I could do it on my own, and that it would be weak of me to admit that I was struggling – what did I have to moan about? On the outside, life was back on track. I was smiling, coping and successful, but inside I felt worthless. Depression – as I now see it for what it was – had pulled its black bag over my head and I was suffocating. It was like drowning on dry land, in full view of the world, but no one knew.

I loved my children so much my heart could burst, but I didn't think I was good enough for them. I felt as if I couldn't do anything right and that they'd be better off without me. I didn't tell anyone about these thoughts because I worried that if I said something I'd be judged, or worse, I'd be deemed an unfit mother and my children would be taken away from me. So I laughed and played and loved them so much they would never have known anything was wrong. But inside I was broken.

One day, after coming off air on *Loose Women* and crying all the way home in the car, I decided I had to do something about how I was feeling. There was a lovely doctor at my local surgery who seemed kind and non-judgemental. During my appointment with her, I broke down and told her everything. She listened, and asked me about what else was going on in my life. I explained the events of the previous few years and she (rightly, I now think) said she thought that I wasn't just postnatally depressed, I was struggling to cope with everything I'd been through.

I now had a new baby with a new partner, and had moved away from the area I'd lived in most of my adult life to start afresh, so I had no support network. I'd gone back to work twelve weeks after giving birth and had started a new job, which was proving tricky. It was enough to make anyone wobble! She put me on antidepressants, and told me to come back and see her again in a few months.

I didn't tell a soul that I was taking the medication. It can be so hard to seek help in the first place, to admit you're getting it is an even bigger issue, and, like the menopause, postnatal depression is something women keep to themselves all too often out of some kind of shame. Which is a shame in itself, because the reality is that when you have a new baby you're under a lot of pressure physically and emotionally, so it's not a great surprise when all is not completely well.

I kept quiet partly because I wanted to see if anyone noticed a difference in me once I started taking the medication, or was this all going on in my head? A month went by and my partner remarked that I seemed to be more cheerful. Another couple of weeks passed and I stopped feeling tearful every day on my way home from work, overwhelmed with feeling like I couldn't do my job and nobody liked me. It was as if a switch had been flicked in my brain, and I could think clearly for the first time in years.

I truly believe that antidepressants helped me get back on track after a very difficult time in my life, and I'm glad I took them. Much like going on HRT, it was an ah-ha moment when I realized that I didn't have to feel the way I did. I could take control and do something about it. I could feel like myself again. I ended up staying on the pills for a few years and decided to wean myself off them in my own time, when I felt ready.

In fact, right at that time, life threw me yet another curve ball, and I found myself on my own again. Many people would reach for the pills following the break-up of a relationship, but I wanted to manage by myself – without the antidepressants. So I slowly reduced how often I was taking them – from every day, to every other day, to a few times a week until, after months of tiny steps, I'd walked away from them fully.

When I was depressed I'd needed the medication to help with an imbalance in my brain, an imbalance that very gradually, and over time, corrected itself. That's not to say I didn't feel pain and sadness once I'd stopped taking the antidepressants – I did – but this time it was very different to the feelings of depression I'd had after the birth of my daughter. These were emotions I was *supposed* to feel, and I let myself – it was part of the process. That's the difference, I think, between depression and the normal sadness and grief there is when a marriage ends.

It was difficult – any life experience such as the one I was going through is bound to be painful – but if I was going to get over it, I needed to feel it in its fullest form, and learn coping strategies. It also meant that when my menopause symptoms kicked in in earnest, I was able to pin down what feeling normal was for *me*, and that's something we can only do as individuals, as although we may all tick off the symptoms on the menopausal checklist, we'll each experience things in our own unique way.

Hot stuff . . . in all the wrong ways

And so it happened that about a year later I noticed a change in my moods again. I was swinging from feeling high and happy to crashingly low and anxious. I was angry a lot of the time and getting increasingly snappy with the kids. None of this was normal. I've always been a pretty steady Eddie and manage to keep a lid on things even during tough times, but I'd started flying off the handle over the smallest thing.

Then, the sweats started again. I've never been a huge sweater – no more than normal, I guess – but over time I noticed that standard antiperspirant wasn't cutting it. I wasn't just sweating under my arms either; it was trickling down my back, around my hairline and my upper lip. At night, I was sweating so much I had to change the sheets almost every day. I could literally wring them out.

These symptoms had first appeared a few years previously

but had gone away. Now they were back with a vengeance. What started as a low, rumbling anxiety, eventually turned into a roar . . .

Keep calm and carry on

For some strange reason, it feels like celebrities aren't expected to go through all this personal stuff. It's as if anyone in the public eye doesn't feel pain or emotion quite like the rest of the world. My mum used to tell me, 'Even the Queen goes to the loo', when I was feeling overawed by someone or something, to remind me that everyone is human. Well, I'm sure that even the Queen has had her hot flushes and moments when she's felt as if the world is against her, but has carried on with the dignity and grace that the world expects of her.

Unlike some women in the public eye, I'm fortunate enough to work in a job where I can talk about my personal experiences, and have been overwhelmed with support from women when I've done so. It hasn't always been this way, though, and I didn't plan to tell the world about my menopause and my decision to have a hysterectomy. It just happened that way.

Have I had a better experience of it because I'm well known? Of course not. My body went through – and is still going through – exactly the same thing as any other woman's. Has it put me under more pressure? That's a difficult one, because all our pressures are different. I'm expected to look professional and act composed at all times, to work through brain fog while keeping everything flowing in front of millions of people on live television; smiling and being charming while I feel anything but. However, isn't everyone expected to grin and bear it? When you're at work, doesn't there have to be at least a veneer of being in control? It's amazing what brilliant actors we become.

The mental struggle against the encroaching menopause is difficult enough, but the physical symptoms can be harder to hide. One minute you're sitting normally, and then you feel a little warm, like someone has turned the heating up, and up, and up . . . The sweat starts to trickle down your neck, armpits, back, upper lip. Ugh, it's horrible. And there's little you can do other than fan yourself and wait for it to pass.

I've been known to wear sanitary towels on every part of my body I could in order to combat the sweats. I've often worn them under my arms to stop the embarrassing sweat circles – I even tried Botox under my arms, which was painful and not a very nice experience at all. It worked, but was too awful to try again!

When my night sweats began to creep into the day, arriving without warning, and normally while I was at work and needing to look my professional best, it was tough. We've all been there – jumping up and down every few minutes to adjust the room temperature, opening and closing windows, and generally getting on everybody's nerves . . . Here's an example of my typical day in a live TV studio, hosting an award-winning show, while in the throes of the menopause. I wrote this on my phone on the way home from work, just a piece of writing about how I'd felt that day . . .

> The sweat was trickling down my back; I could feel it running from the nape of my neck down between my shoulder blades and over the knobbles of my spine. My hairline was sprinkled with pearls of moisture, plastering my expertly curled and sprayed hair to my studio-

strength make-up. I smiled brightly at camera four, and told the million people watching me from home that we'd be back right after the break, my eyes twinkling as I waved them off to the adverts.

Within seconds, the *Loose Women* make-up team descended on the set like a swarm of paratroopers; their arsenal consisting of eyeshadow, lip gloss and tissues to blot our shiny faces and keep us looking our glossy, on-camera best.

Gemma the wardrobe stylist looked at me and I pulled a rueful face as I checked my notes for the next part of the show, listened through my earpiece to my producer talking through her interview thoughts on our next guest, and nodded to show our studio director that I'd heard the instruction to look at camera seven as we came back on air.

I expertly whipped out the two panty liners that had been stuck under my armpits and swapped them for the fresh ones Gemma handed to me, then we both checked to make sure I was sweat-patch free. We smiled at each other and rolled our eyes knowingly – it might look glamorous to the viewers at home, but if only they knew what it took to keep a menopausal woman together during a live TV show.

Within minutes the hot flush had come and gone, and thankfully I was now fresh and ready to get on with the show. Literally . . .

That may be what my day is like for one hour out of twenty-four, but the rest of the time my life is like that of any other menopausal woman, and I'm still fending off sweats and brain fog at the very moment I need them least. That's why

I sometimes think the best thing we can all do when the going gets tough is to channel our inner Elizabeth Taylor and get on with things, but be fabulous while we're at it. As Liz herself said, 'Pour yourself a drink, put on some lipstick and pull yourself together.' Maybe leave out the drink if you're struggling at breakfast time, but you know what I mean.

Good old Liz was also quoted as saying that on some days she, like all of us, had to force herself to get up, to put one foot in front of the other and refuse to let life get to her. She had a point. We're going through this anyway. Why not turn your gritted teeth into a 'sod them all' smile?

While the menopause itself certainly wasn't mentioned in the early days of Hollywood, stars of both the small and big screens have been far more open about their experiences in recent times, with *Baywatch*'s Pamela Anderson telling *Hello!* magazine about her menopause symptoms. She told the magazine in its 6 February 2018 edition that she was apprehensive about it because her mother had had a particularly difficult time, but was open about her physical and emotional changes: 'Hormones! Hot flushes! Moods! I knew something was changing. I definitely feel a change. I think I am perimenopausal, or whatever it is called. I felt very emotional, poetic, very dark and dreamy.'

The actress Kim Cattrall went further in the *Telegraph* (27 February 2018), describing in vivid and all-too-familiar detail her experience of the menopause.

> Literally one moment you're fine, and then another, you feel like you're in a vat of boiling water, and you feel like the rug has been pulled from beneath you ... What I would say, which I've said to myself and to girlfriends who've also

experienced hot flashes, in particular, is that change is part of being human. We evolve and should not fear that change. You're not alone. I feel that part of living this long is experiencing this, so I'm trying to turn it into a very positive thing for myself, which it has been, in the sense of acceptance and tolerance and education about this time of life.

When female stars renowned for their youth and beauty start 'confessing' about their experiences of the menopause – that taboo word so synonymous with ageing – you know that times are changing. And this, I think we can all agree, is fantastic news for all of us!

Dr Peers Says . . .

ENDOMETRIOSIS

Endometriosis is a chronic and painful condition caused when fragments of the cells lining the womb, called the endometrium, are found elsewhere in the body. During the menstrual cycle, these cell fragments grow and can cause severe pain. Eventually, the fragments break down and bleed but, unlike the lining that is shed during your period, they can't leave the body. They cause inflammation, pain and scar tissue, known as adhesions, and can lead to infertility, fatigue, and bowel and bladder problems.

Such symptoms are not exclusive to endometriosis and so reaching a diagnosis can take a long time. A laparoscopy is the best way to diagnose the condition. It involves a small camera – a laparoscope – being inserted into the body through a small cut near the navel. If endometriosis is detected, it can either be treated at the same time, using laparoscopic surgery, or the tissue can be removed for further investigation. Laparoscopic keyhole surgery leaves minimal scars and has a rapid post-operative recovery time.[1]

POSTNATAL DEPRESSION

Around 10 to 15 per cent of new mothers experience postnatal depression (PND). It usually develops within six weeks of giving birth. It can make you feel hopeless about the future, tearful for no apparent reason as well as tired and unable to cope. Whilst it's easy to blame hormones at this time – and they can trigger changes in mood – there are many other factors that also play a part in the development of the condition. These include previous episodes of depression, lack of support from family or friends, or recent experience of a stressful or upsetting life event, such as bereavement or the end of a relationship. For some women, there may be a physical cause for their depression: for example, an underactive thyroid, which can be easily treated. It's a condition we should all be aware of and we should be vigilant to help our friends and daughters if we suspect they're suffering.[2]

1 Sources: Endometriosis UK. Understanding endometriosis. www.endometriosis-uk.org/understanding-endometriosis; Endometriosis UK. Getting diagnosed with endometriosis. www.endometriosis-uk.org/getting-diagnosed-endometriosis

2 Sources: www.rcpsych.ac.uk/healthadvice/problemsanddisorders/postnataldepression.aspx; MIND fact sheet

3

Serious Lady Bit Problems

....

'Aged thirty-six, had a total hysterectomy three years ago, on HRT, been off work with stress. It's so hard.'

'The hysterectomy was a last resort to ease the pain after eight surgeries over ten years . . .'

'Been a nightmare for five years after hysterectomy, but have found progesterone cream, which has been a miracle.'

'I had a hysterectomy seven years ago (aged thirty-five). I didn't launch into the menopause but I certainly felt an end to certain aspects of womanhood. Maybe I'm saying it wrong, but I felt as if I did go through "an ending".'

....

My decision to have a hysterectomy at the age of forty-six didn't happen overnight, but it seemed to be the logical choice based on what was happening to me at the time. Once I'd made my choice, I started looking into what I could do to prepare myself for it – in every way. Mentally, physically and emotionally I needed to know that I was doing the right things to keep me on track.

I started reading up on what it would mean to have my reproductive organs removed. I did what we all do when presented with something we don't fully understand: I went straight to Google. If you're reading this book, then there's a big chance you've also done the same thing – terrifying, isn't it? There's so much *stuff* out there, on all sorts of websites; from medical ones that list every possible complication, to forums sharing horror stories that make your hair curl. My advice? Stick to legitimate sources, such as NHS Choices, so you know that the information you're being given is solid.

A hysterectomy to remove my womb and ovaries would hopefully end years of pain as a result of endometriosis and ovarian cysts. None of the various operations I'd had in the past had been much fun, but they'd been necessary to fix physical problems with my body that were causing pain and were potentially harmful.

My biggest fear wasn't the hysterectomy itself; it was that I'd go mad afterwards. I knew having an operation wouldn't be pleasant – it's always taken me for ever to cope with the after-effects of anaesthetic, so the first few weeks were always going to be bumpy, physically speaking – but I'd never had surgery that could have a profound effect on my mental health. That's what was making me nervous about it, and I think this gets to the heart of one of the key issues with the menopause. It's tough from a physical point of view, but we manage to find a way to deal with that – we *are* tough. We are strong. However, when things get difficult mentally, that can be where the real problem lies.

My life was finally good by this point. Things had fallen into place for me professionally and personally, and I didn't want to do anything that might jeopardize my happiness. I felt content, and the only fly in the ointment was the pain I was contending with on a daily basis, and which was increasing.

It wasn't just the dull, throbbing pain in my lower left side that seemed to have been there for ever, it was now sharp and stabbing, sometimes leaving me curled up and tearful, gulping down paracetamol and willing it to pass. Should I just deal with it, like I'd always done – and like most women with endometriosis do – and simply carry on? Or should I take the plunge and do something about it?

Why a hysterectomy?

I had a series of tests done to rule out any other possible causes of the pain I was in. It turned out that my left kidney was enlarged and the veins running from it to my bladder had become varicose, which was probably causing some of my pain, but not all of it.

My urologist recommended that I meet Mr Jan, a gynaecologist who specializes in endometriosis. I did, and we decided I should have a laparoscopy (again) to see what was happening. It was originally booked for around Christmas 2015 but then, as the time got nearer, I became busy with work and so I rescheduled for the new year. Then, out of the blue, I had my first period in about seven years.

I'd had a Mirena coil fitted, which had been helping with my endometriosis by pumping hormones into my pelvic area whilst also acting as birth control. Once it was in I didn't have to think about it, and since I'd had it my periods had stopped. As I was also on a low dose of HRT for the perimenopause, periods were completely off my radar, so its arrival took me completely by surprise.

It was awful. The bleeding lasted for weeks, and I was in constant agony. I went back to see Mr Jan, and we came to the conclusion that there was little point in having one operation to have a look around, then another one to fix what might be wrong, when it was pretty obvious that things weren't working too well in there. We agreed to proceed with a hysterectomy, get it all out and hopefully be pain-free.

I was nervously happy about this decision, if that makes sense. I was content with the two wonderful children I had, and wasn't planning on having any more. I was already starting the menopause and would be looking into managing it over the coming years, so the decision made practical sense. Even if it was a scary one.

Menopause: to discuss or not to discuss?

I didn't intend to talk publicly about going through the menopause, but here we are. Nor did I think I'd end up telling the world about my hysterectomy. I was hesitant for a couple of reasons: I didn't feel like it was anyone else's business, and I also didn't want people to think I was over the hill. That old chestnut.

So how *did* it all end up coming out? Well, it was thanks to my friend Linda 'Baggy Mouth' Robson, the lovely *Loose Women* panellist and actress of *Birds of a Feather* fame. I was at work with my colleagues, who all knew that I was due to have my operation the following day and was going to need a month off work to recover. We'd talked about it several months previously as I'd been booked in for surgery three months earlier, but had had to cancel because of work commitments. They knew how nervous I was.

One thing I *hadn't* given any thought to was what I was going to tell the loyal *Loose Women* viewers. In my head, I was simply going to leave quietly and have my operation, take a month off to get well and come back to work. My family, friends, colleagues and bosses knew what was happening, and that was all I thought I needed to take care of.

Then, Linda piped up in the morning meeting, 'You'll need to tell people something, Andrea, or they'll all think you've been fired!'

Well . . . that hadn't crossed my mind at all! But she was right. Telling your boss and your colleagues is a difficult enough thing to consider when you have a personal issue, such as dealing with time off to recover from a sensitive operation. I work in a job where I had to think about what the public, and also the press, might think as well – left to their own imaginations, all sorts of reasons might be conjured up as to why I wasn't at work.

This is something I've heard many times from women: no matter what your job is, telling the people you work for, or with, that you're going to have a life-changing operation is scary. How will they react? Will they be supportive, or will you now have one more thing to worry about while you're off recovering?

Talking in the workplace about the menopause, including hysterectomies, is still incredibly difficult, and many women choose not to do it for a number of reasons: they don't want to be stigmatized by their bosses or peers, they worry they might not be seen to be as capable of doing their job, or they simply feel it's a personal issue that they'd rather not share. In a recent 2017 survey conducted by research consultancy ComRes for Radio Sheffield and Radio 4's *Woman's Hour*, 70 per cent of women did not tell their employers that they were experiencing menopause symptoms, despite almost half of them saying they felt those symptoms affected their mental health.

Some workplaces are taking steps to introduce their own menopause policy, including Nottinghamshire Police, thanks to the work of former chief constable Sue Fish, who was horrified to discover that talented, experienced women were leaving the force early because of the severity of their symptoms and lack of support.

In February 2018 it was revealed by the Office for National Statistics that the number of working women aged fifty or over had hit a record high of 4.7 million. With the female retirement age due to rise this year to sixty-five, older women in the workforce is a reality that employers have to face, and deal with.

Having a menopause policy as standard in any workplace would mean that managers have guidelines to follow and women would know they are supported – just as they would if they were pregnant or going through any other health issue. It would mean menopause-related problems such as migraines, difficulties with decision-making, memory lapses, depression and irritability can be managed, not ignored and not used to stigmatize people. Normalizing menopause in society's eyes means changing the attitudes, perceptions and behaviour of people in every corner of a woman's life, be it partners, GPs or work colleagues who, whether through lack of information or otherwise, can be unenlightened and unsupportive.

Little things mean a lot at work. Just knowing that you can have a fan at your desk; change where you sit so that you're by a window; start slightly later in the day, perhaps, to allow for sleep deprivation; have the flexibility to work at home more; or have time off for medical appointments – these are simple things that don't cost anything, but can make a huge difference. It's all about creating a new work culture. Good ventilation, blinds, cold drinking water, workplace rest areas or lighter, non-synthetic uniforms (where relevant) are all things employers could consider.

When the time came to make my own announcement I was apprehensive as we went on air. I knew I had to say something about the fact that I was having time off, but I didn't know what to say, or when to say it. I needn't have worried. Linda Robson took control! As we came to the end of the show, I still hadn't mentioned it. She interrupted our final conversation, looked me in the eye and said, 'Before we finish that, Andrea, you're not going to be with us for the next few weeks, are you? We're going to miss you . . .'

My stomach dropped to the floor because I knew what she was doing; she was making sure I didn't do what I normally do when there's something I don't want to say on the show . . . I allow everyone else to talk, let the time slide away, and then move on without putting my opinion into the mix. She wasn't letting me get away with that this time!

My heart began to pound, although I sounded fairly calm on the telly (I've watched the footage back and I don't think you can tell that I felt as if I was either going to cry or throw up). I simply said, 'Just to let you know, don't worry if you don't see me for the next month or so, I'm actually going to be off at home convalescing. I'm having a hysterectomy tomorrow. Lots of personal reasons for that. I did go to the doctors and talk about it!' We'd been talking earlier on the show about going to your doctor about health worries.

Saira Khan jumped up and gave me a big hug, which nearly

set me off, but I ploughed on, heart thumping and doing my best to look like a capable TV host rather than betray what I actually was – a really scared woman telling the world that she was about to have a life-changing operation. Inside, I was a quivering wreck.

'You'll be all right, you'll be all right . . .' Saira said, as she cuddled me. I couldn't look at her because I knew I'd cry.

'Um, so, yeah . . .' I continued. 'I will be at home watching you guys. I may be tweeting in . . . but that's where I'm going to be, just in case you were wondering.'

Apart from when I stumbled over the word 'hysterectomy' (it almost sounds like I'm having an hysterical-ectomy – which is about right!), you wouldn't know that inside I was a mess. I was trying with all my might to hold myself together, not to fall apart. Saying it out loud had made it *real*. I was actually doing this, I couldn't back out now! And this is what so many of us do – pretend it's not happening, that it's all OK, keep that stiff upper lip firmly in place. We've got to stop doing that.

The Loose Women could not have been nicer. The team that we have now is the best it's been for years. There is genuine friendship, love and laughter off set, as well as the banter and disagreement that you see when we go live. We're friends; and that's why we're able to be as honest as we are, because we know we can trust each other. No one's going to stitch you up and say something on the telly that you've confided in private; we've got each other's backs.

You'll have a group of mates you love and trust, too, I hope. It makes all the difference. It's so important to talk about how you're feeling with friends you're comfortable with. Scary things like operations can become even more frightening if we let them fester in our heads, and I for one am known to let things grow to unmanageable proportions by keeping them in. Let them out. Talk. Share. Don't work yourself up into a lather, because the reality is rarely as bad as we think it's going to be. And if it is, you have friends you can lean on, so use them . . . After all, as the song goes, isn't that what they're for?

D-Day: No going back

The day you wake up knowing you're going to have the essence of your womanhood removed is never going to be an easy one, and the feelings of fear and loss are difficult to sum up in words. So many of you have experienced this, too, as I know from the messages I've received.

The alarm went off at 6 a.m. and I lay in the dark, letting myself slowly come to. This was it. I got up and showered with the horrible-smelling pink cleanser the hospital had given me to ward off MRSA, washing my hair in it for hopefully the last time. It was strange getting dressed in my baggiest tracksuit bottoms and sweatshirt, no make-up on, roughly dried hair, and thinking, 'Right, that's me ready to go . . .' It felt as if I was going on a really rubbish holiday. I checked my bag and made sure I had everything I needed for my hospital stay. My husband, Nick, was up, showered and dressed too, and when our brilliant mother's help, Lin, arrived at 7 a.m. to take over with the kids, we were ready to leave.

My son, Fin, was in the shower, and I didn't want to make a fuss and ask him to come out just to hug his mum goodbye, so I shouted through the door, 'Bye, Fin. I'm heading off now. See you later!' Just like it was any other work day.

'Bye, Mum. See you later!' came the reply. Like a typical

fourteen-year-old boy; I wasn't sure he even remembered I was heading to the hospital.

My daughter, Amy, gave me a big squeeze as we headed to the door. 'Bye, Mum. We'll come and see you in hospital.' Lin hugged me too, and told me it would all be fine. I pretended I believed her. I headed to the car with Nick, handbag and overnight bag in hand.

We reached the hospital in five minutes; it was that close to our house. It made it feel all the more surreal: the kids were just down the road at home, getting ready for a normal school day, and I was walking into hospital, getting ready for God knows what.

Nick and I were shown to my room, and I was told to get into my hospital gown. Nurses came and went, checking my name and details over and over again. The anaesthetist and then my surgeon, Mr Jan, arrived, checking my details again, and giving me the chance to ask any last-minute questions. I didn't have any – I couldn't really think straight, if I'm honest. I wondered if all these people were popping in constantly just in case I was thinking of running away. Maybe they've seen that happen. It certainly crossed my mind, even though I'd be fleeing in my hospital gown, bum bouncing for all the world to see . . .

I was the first operation of the day, which was great news, as I had less chance to think. In no time at all, I was being asked to make my way down to theatre. This was it. Nick and I looked at each other with fear in our eyes for the first time. We'd kept things light-hearted and chatty all morning, but in an instant it all changed. He stood up and hugged me before we left the room, and I could see he had tears in his eyes.

'It'll be fine,' he said, but I think he was reassuring himself as much as me. We walked hand in hand, following a male nurse bedecked in scrubs and rubber surgical clogs into the lift, and stood in silence as it gently lowered us to the floor below. As we got out, Nick stood and watched as I walked away from him, down the long white corridor to the surgical suite. I turned back to see him wave, and gave him a little one in return. The nurse was a big man, and he walked faster than me down the hallway. The floor was cold under my bare feet – I'd forgotten my slippers.

'I feel like I'm being led to the electric chair,' I joked weakly, fighting back tears. Now that Nick was gone, I didn't have to be brave for anyone any more.

He laughed. 'Ah, yes, we call it the Green Mile.'

'That's not helping . . .' I thought to myself.

By the time I got to the pre-med room, I was gulping back tears. I was glad it wasn't the actual operating theatre, and was just a small room to the side where I'd be sent to sleep gently. I'd have been even more terrified if I'd seen the table, the lights and the surgical instruments . . . The anaesthetist was waiting for me by the bed. She was a tall, attractive blonde woman, who looked capable and kind. I smiled and said hello as I climbed up, taking care not to flash anyone as my hospital gown gaped open at the back.

'How are you feeling?' she asked me. I looked up at her and my veneer of bravery dropped away. I'd held it together for the kids before I'd left home that morning, and for Nick, but now it was just me, I couldn't. My usual, cheerful, stiff upper lip betrayed me, and it wobbled as the words tumbled out.

'I'm really scared.' Such small words that didn't come close to describing the monster-sized fear that was welling up inside me. I felt as if I was being swallowed up from the inside out.

'I don't want to wait,' I said, tears trickling out of my eyes and into my ears as I lay flat. 'Please just knock me out now, so I don't have to think about this any more.'

Even as I spoke, fear and nausea choked the words in my mouth.

The anaesthetist gently inserted a long needle into one of the veins on the back of my hand, and strapped a tube to it. As she expertly connected it to the drugs that would soon send me to sleep, she asked me if I'd been on holiday that year. I was confused – why was she asking me about holidays now? The polite, good girl in me replied yes, I'd had a quick break to Mykonos with Nick.

'Well, imagine you're in Mykonos.' She smiled. 'You're watching a lovely sunset and are about to have a nice, long, cool gin and tonic.'

My mind flashed to the holiday, and an evening out we'd had with my *Loose Women* friend Jane Moore, whom we'd bumped into at the airport. We had indeed gone for a sundowner together, and the image sprang into my anxious mind.

'You should feel something cold coming into you now,' the anaesthetist said, and there it was, the beginnings of the very drug I was so afraid of and so longed for. 'As you feel it going up your arm, imagine you're watching that beautiful sunset, you're warm and relaxed, and that cool gin and tonic is just hitting the spot . . .'

She may have said more, but as the image of me and Jane Moore having a sundowner faded before my eyes, I had one last jolt of panic. What would happen to me while I was asleep? And worse, would I ever be the same again once I'd woken up?

A fresh start

It was about three hours later when I finally came round. I was back in my room, in my bed. I could hear someone saying my name, over and over again, telling me to wake up. I felt as if I was at the bottom of a dark pit and the voice was far away, getting closer and louder each time. I slowly opened my eyes. A nurse was standing over me, telling me that I was back from the operation and it had all gone well. Mr Jan was happy, and would be in shortly to talk me through it. I closed my eyes again and let myself drift away. It was done.

The rest of the day was a haze of sleeping and feeling horribly, horrendously sick. I couldn't stay awake. I couldn't eat any food that was offered to me to help quell the nausea, as I had no saliva in my mouth. It took me hours to chew one piece of toast, as I kept falling asleep with it in my mouth – a dry, squashed ball of mush that I couldn't swallow, so it lay lodged inside my cheek as I drifted in and out of consciousness.

I wasn't in any real pain. I felt strange – aware but not aware of what was happening to me and around me – but I did have an overwhelming sensation of nausea, which blocked out everything else. Amy and Lin came to visit me after school, but I kept nodding off. I knew it must have been a bit frightening for Amy, so I tried to be as normal and smiley as I could, but I'm sure my pale face, the tubes coming out of me, and the fact that I kept drifting away every few minutes must have been unsettling for her.

Mr Jan came in to see me at one point and told me about the operation. I couldn't remember most of what he said, apart from that he'd had to stitch my bladder, and that my bowel had been stuck to the mesh of my old hernia repair, so he'd had to move and stitch that up too. It sounded gruesome.

A few hours later Nick arrived, having driven to Birmingham and back in the time since I'd waved him goodbye. How strange that my life had changed for ever during those few hours that the children had been at school and he'd been at work. What a strange parallel our lives had run in. We both got a little tearful, him when he saw me in bed, and me when I saw his kind, concerned face. When the time came for him to leave, I didn't want him to go, but I also didn't want him to see me as I was. I hoped I'd be a bit better in the morning . . .

First-night blues

The night following the operation was one of the worst I have ever known. It lasted for ever, and was a dark night of pain, nausea and light-headedness. My blood pressure dropped through the floor, and I had to be tipped back in my bed to raise my legs higher than my head. I felt as if I was on the world's slowest and least fun rollercoaster.

The worst of the pain came from the after-effects of the gas that had been pumped into my abdomen during the operation so the surgeon could see what he was doing, while disconnecting my womb, fallopian tubes, ovaries and cervix through three laparoscopic holes and removing them through my vagina. Some of the air was still trapped in my body. I was in complete and utter agony. I was given liquid morphine to drink, an anti-nausea tablet, a paracetamol drip and ibuprofen capsules, which took the edge off but didn't totally relieve me of my symptoms.

I thought the night would never end. The only thing that

made it bearable was the lovely nurse called Dawn, who, true to her name, looked after me until the sun rose the next day.

Partly to help with the anxiety I was experiencing, I kept a diary of what happened to me in the month following my hysterectomy. It's very raw and gets across what I was going through at the time. So this is what I wrote, pretty much word for word.

Day 1

Agony. All day. Trapped air in my stomach, shoulder pain. Fuzzy-headed. My catheter is removed, which feels horrible even though the nurse, Lin, did it as nicely as she could. She wipes me down while telling me she watches me on telly, which is embarrassing.

Another nurse, chatty and bubbly, tells me about her life in Japan and Hong Kong as an expat. She lets Nick guide me to the bathroom and he showers me as I sit pathetically on a plastic chair. He's so gentle and loving I want to cry, but I feel too sick. The nurse points out it's because my bladder and bowels have been moved and touched, and they're not happy about it. Neither am I.

I spend the rest of the day in a granny chair in my room, or sleeping. The trapped air is horrendous. I have morphine syrup spoon-fed to me like a child. It makes me feel sleepy but sick, and I don't know what's worse.

Day 2

The nurse gives me laxative syrup, which makes no difference. Then she gives me suppositories and the rumbling starts. It's horrifying, having no control over my body. The wind starts to come out, but I'm frightened to let it in case I poo myself, because that's what it feels like is going to happen. I spend the day shuffling back and forth to the toilet and trumping painfully as the air finally makes its way out of my body. I feel sick from the codeine, but the pain is so bad it's taking my breath away.

There aren't as many staff on as it's a Saturday. I feel abandoned – one jug of water all day, had to ask for some crackers as I was hungry. Managed a shower on my own. Ask for a hairdryer, rude girl behind the desk makes me feel like a pain in the neck for asking and I get tearful about it, and cross that I'm not strong enough to stick up for myself. I decide to go home that night – I've had enough. Nick picks me up with the kids, I really hope no paps have got a picture of me. I look horrendous.

When I get home I lie on the couch on our porch under a throw. My happy place. *Loose Women* have asked me to make a little film for the viewers, saying thank you for their messages, so Nick films me as I'm lying there and I send it in.

Mum and Dad come and see me, straight over after getting back from their golden-wedding-anniversary trip round Scotland. The kids, Nick and I start watching *The Time Traveler's Wife*, but I can't make sense of it at all, so I go to bed.

My first night back home, it's strange. I can't do my normal things. I have to sleep half upright in my own bed, and I'm scared of keeping Nick awake. I manage to sleep until 4.30 a.m. before the pain creeps in.

Day 3

The day passes in a haze of pain and sleep. I lie outside on the porch for most of it, getting fresh air when I can, wrapped up in a throw. The trapped air is still causing me the most pain – it brings tears to my eyes – and I'm still frightened every time I think any is coming out, so I can't help but hold it in, even though I know it's the worst thing I can do. The painkillers are taking away the worst of the pain from the operation, but this is a killer.

Day 4

I wake up at 4.30 again with pain in my back as well as my stomach. My bed is obviously too soft to be sleeping like I am, propped up with pillows. I lie still until 5.30 and Nick's alarm goes off; he has to take the girls back to Eastbourne where they live. I don't want to risk waking him and have him lose a precious hour's sleep.

I manage to get back to sleep until about 10 a.m., when I hear Lin moving around. She hadn't wanted to leave me on my own while Nick is out of the house. I tell her it's OK to go, and shuffle about. I want to make every day a productive day, so that I don't feel useless. I want to achieve something each day, even if it's only a small thing.

I tell Lin I won't have a shower until Nick is home, but I do. I put on a face pack and pluck my eyebrows, things I usually rush because I don't have time. I now have all the time. I put a little make-up on. I don't want to look like a hundred-year-old nana, it makes me feel worse.

I feel OK today, though. A bit groggy in the head, but better. The pain in my stomach is gradually lessening; the laxatives are starting to bring me back to normal, and I can't describe the relief that brings, to finally go to the toilet. You probably wouldn't want me to either, but you know what I mean.

Mid-afternoon I get jittery because I haven't written my column yet for the *Mirror*. It's due tomorrow. It takes me for ever because my mind keeps fuzzing over, then the pain kicks in, but I manage to get it done and sent. That's my achievement for the day, so I'm pleased.

I spend the rest of the early evening watching the film *The Secret Garden* with Amy as she's doing it at school, and we've been reading *Return to the Secret Garden* as her bedtime story. She snuggles into me under the throw and it's nice. A couple of *Modern Family*s later and it's bedtime. Then Nick and I catch up with *Cold Feet* and it's time for bed. I think I'm going to be watching a *lot* of TV.

Day 5

I wake at 5 a.m. and try to get comfortable in bed but I can't. And then I hear a squeak. Is that a mouse? How can we have a mouse? I wait for the noise to come again. There! A squeak! It's coming from my right – is it on the floor? Oh God, is it climbing up the curtains? Or worse, on to the bed? I freeze, my already-sore back groaning silently. This time the squeak comes with a clicking sound. Since when did mice click?

I strain my ears, concentrating in the dark. *Squeak. Click. Sigh* . . . The mattress sinks to my side as Nick takes a long deep breath and, by the sound and movement of things, rolls on to his side. Another long sigh . . . and then silence.

Either the mouse is frozen to the curtain – as I am to the side of the bed, waiting for Nick to settle – or, and I slowly realize that this is the more likely answer, the noises I've heard have come from him. He's not snoring . . . he's squeaking in his sleep! How have I never noticed this before?

I stare into the darkness, wondering what time it is. I'm now wide awake. It's Night 5 following my operation, and I'm still not used to sleeping on my back, half propped up by pillows – two under my head and shoulders, and one under my knees. It's my second night without codeine, and my third without morphine, so it stands to reason that pain will be poking me awake at some point.

I feel in the dark for my phone charging on my bedside table, hoping the light won't wake Nick. The time glares out at me – 5.20 a.m. That isn't bad at all. It means I've managed almost six hours of full sleep, my longest stretch yet. But after lying awake for what feels like an eternity, I need painkillers, a wee, and to stretch my aching back. I ease myself up as quietly as I can, my teeth gritted with effort. I slide my hospital-stockinged feet into my slippers and pull on my dressing gown. The door handle makes its familiar squeak as I try to creep out of the room.

Nick stirs and mumbles, 'You OK?'

'I'm fine,' I whisper. 'Go back to sleep.'

I think he's out by the time I reach the bottom of the stairs.

Jackson, our dog, wags his tail as I pad slowly towards him, happy to see anyone at this time of day. I let him out the back door to bark into the darkness, and make myself a cup of herbal tea.

I don't want this to become my new normal. I like

sleeping and 5.20 is way too early for me to be getting up if there isn't work or a holiday flight calling. I open my laptop to start writing, and I'm still sitting there when Fin walks in and looks surprised to see me. He's already up, showered and dressed for school, walking round with his headphones in like he usually does.

At 7.45 Amy still hasn't surfaced. This is very unusual – I'd expected her to be sitting downstairs when I got there. She is *always* up first. I head upstairs and open her blinds quietly, letting the light wake her. It's so rare to get the chance to wake Amy up – she's been up before all of us since the day she was born. In the past few years she's been old enough to take care of herself in the mornings, so I've left her to it until I've been needed to do the last bits before she's ready for school: teeth brushed, hair done, bag packed and ready to go.

'Amy,' I say quietly, 'it's time to get up.'

She rolls on to her back, screwing her face up at the unwelcome light.

'Morning . . . You've had a bit of a lie-in.' I speak quietly. One of my pet hates is being rudely awakened, so I never do it to anyone else. My wake-up calls are always gentle and slow. Anyone who thinks of yanking the covers off, flinging open the curtains and yelling, 'Time to get up!' will find themselves getting short shrift from me. And possibly a black eye . . . Mornings are for coming round slowly, not being blasted into consciousness.

I move her hair off her hot face and smile down at her.

The rest of the day passed. I tried to go back to bed to catch up on sleep, but I couldn't nod off, so I gave up and

got showered and dressed. Mum came over with her
infamous chicken and vegetable soup for me, and stayed
for a few hours, catching up on stuff.

We watched *Loose Women* together as we ate our lunch,
and I was horrified when they played the little film I'd sent
them a few days ago. Oh my God. I looked about 104. Pale
and quiet, lying on the sofa on the porch with a throw over
me, my hands tucked under my chin like Little Red Riding
Hood's granny. All I needed was the bonnet. Coleen was
hosting, and I nearly spat out my soup when she announced
that over *ten thousand* viewers had been in touch with the
show to wish me well. Tears sprang to my eyes.

By the end of the day, Dad had popped round to put
up some pictures, Nick was back and telling me excitedly
about the garden centres he'd visited to ask about putting
up one of his garden pods, and his plans for the exhibition
at the NEC he was doing in six weeks. Lin had brought
Amy home, then taken her off to gymnastics, and I'd not
left the sofa.

I was desperate for a walk. I needed to get out of the
house and stretch my legs, so Nick took me to the end of the
road and back again, with me clinging on and shuffling next
to him. I was so scared of tripping on the uneven pavement
and jolting myself that I was walking stiffly and unnaturally.

'You're going to make it worse,' he warned me. By the
time we got back to the house I was sore.

I'd stupidly decided that I felt OK, so after my painkillers first thing this morning, I hadn't taken any more.
I thought I'd see if I felt clearer-headed without them.
What I hadn't realized was I obviously still had some in
my system, and they'd been carrying me through the day.

By early evening, the last drop of pain relief left my body, and it was like falling off a cliff. I felt as if I'd been kicked in the abdomen and groin by a horse. A very, very big, angry horse.

I threw paracetamol and ibuprofen down my throat and willed it to work. As I crouched on the little stool by Amy's bed, reading her bedtime story, I struggled to concentrate. I settled her down, said goodnight to Fin – after listening to a particularly obnoxious-sounding prank on his favourite show *Impractical Jokers* and pretending to find it funny – then went back downstairs.

Nick was busy texting and looking up stuff for his exhibition, so I watched some telly, then we made our way to bed. By then the painkillers had started to kick in. Hopefully, after my early start, I'll finally get a full night's sleep.

Day 6

Is it Day 6, or Day 5½ going horribly wrong? I woke at 1.30 a.m. with a start. Wide awake. The painkillers had worn off again, so I got up, went to the loo, took some pills and tried to settle back to sleep. I couldn't get comfortable.

My muscles are starting to scream from lack of use; I'm usually running round all day, walking, lifting, stretching. They're not used to this level of inactivity, and I can feel them losing their strength already, and they're twitching in protest. By now I'd have been to the gym at least once this week, or done some kind of exercise, and my body and brain don't like it at all.

I can feel myself shifting uncomfortably next to Nick

and I don't want to wake him, so at 2 a.m. I'm sitting downstairs in the kitchen, dog at my feet, writing this. I don't know what else to do. I write until 4.45 a.m., have a bowl of Weetabix with banana until 5, and manage to creep back into bed without waking Nick. Bloody hell. This really is the hard bit.

(Also: my sense of smell has suddenly become supersonic, like it was when I was pregnant. The whiff of rotting food in the bin nearly made me keel over, and I can smell people's body odour, their hair, perfume and aftershave like I couldn't before. Is this a side effect?)

I slept on and off until 10 a.m. and was woken by Nick checking on me. I need to get our squeaky door handle fixed. It could wake the dead. I told him about my night, and he checked his sleep app . . . Yup, 100 per cent sleep for him, second night on the trot. The swine.

Day 7

Took some Nytol last night. Managed an almost full night – up a few times. A very productive day sitting outside on the porch, wrapped in a fluffy throw. My parents came to visit, then we spent a quiet night watching the *Steve Jobs* film with Michael Fassbender and Kate Winslet. It was very good.

Felt better today keeping on top of the painkillers – I will *not* be making that mistake again! I even had a glass of red wine, which went down very well. I don't know if I'm allowed to have that yet, but damn it was good! With that and my Nytol, fingers crossed for a full night's sleep.

Day 8

I managed to sleep until 6.30 a.m.! Whoop whoop! My best yet. Got up and dressed, and even managed a short walk. It was a lovely day of sunshine and showers, but with a chill in the air, so I stayed in, wrapped up and focused on my writing while Nick worked at the kitchen table. A quiet day, then caught up on telly programmes I'd recorded – namely the start of a *Ray Donovan* marathon!

Day 9

We took Jackson out for a walk as we were all getting cabin fever, and managed to get absolutely *drenched* in a sudden shower of epic proportions. I swear it wouldn't have looked real if you saw it on telly. We ducked into a nearby pub and tucked into some crisps and a glass of wine while we dried off. Another quiet night, where we both stayed up way too late watching *Ray*. I had two more cheeky glasses of wine, because the first one tasted so nice . . .

Day 10

Woke up at 9.30 and it was as if I'd had a wild night out. I felt dreadful – how can three glasses of wine do this? I lay on the sofa until mid-afternoon, eating bacon sandwiches and watching TV, feeling like a useless teenager.

I finally got to take off my surgical stockings and my plasters! I was very happy about the stockings, because aside from looking horrible they made me really hot at night. I'm sure they were one of the (many) reasons I wasn't sleeping well.

I took the plasters off after my shower. I was nervous – what would my scars look like? There were four small incisions: one up by my ribs on my left side, and three running from hip to hip above another line, thin at the ends but dark and stretched in the middle, from previous abdominal repairs for multiple hernias and two emergency C-sections. My stomach looked like a battlefield of surgery scars. I don't have a real belly button either; I have a scarred hole where one umbilical hernia was repaired. Added to that, I have what look like four gunshot wounds. All my scars are the result of problems that have come from emergency births, damaged muscles, hernias and endometriosis.

I stood in front of the bathroom mirror and studied myself. The wounds were dark and scabbed, but small compared to the war zone under the skin. That itself looked puckered in places, from being stretched and pulled in pregnancy and surgery, and would never sit smooth and taut again.

Little dimples of cellulite were dotted across it, and it felt odd if I touched it. It was as if all the nerve endings from below my breasts down to my groin had been cut. This wasn't anything new – my stomach had looked and felt like this for years – so another few new scars didn't make any difference to me. I stared at them, and asked myself how I felt.

I felt relieved. Hopefully, this was the end of it. No more pain, no more surgery. A fresh start. I felt good.

Day 11

An early awakening again at 6.30 a.m. Amy was very excited about her school project, which, for some reason, she'd decided to work on this morning. It was to do with family fingerprints and we all had to help with it. Fin was oblivious to us all, did his chores and headed off to school, headphones in, music roaring in his ears.

I wrote my column, then at lunchtime Nick suggested we try to walk into town. It was a crisp, bright October day, so why not? I didn't realize how slowly I was moving until I clocked that I was permanently lagging behind Nick, like an obedient wife. I was having none of that, so I asked him to slow down. We laughed as we both realized we hadn't walked that slowly since we had toddlers. I wasn't stopping to examine every snail and point at ants, and although I was tired, I wasn't about to lie on the floor and scream until I was picked up, so it was all good.

Day 12

I slept all the way through until 7 a.m.! I'd tried Kalms Night tablets and they seemed to work better than Nytol for me. Apart from waking up to roll over carefully, I'd had the best night's sleep yet.

I worked for a while in the morning, then prepared lunch for Linda Robson and Nadia Sawalha, who were coming round to visit. I made soup, then fresh bread in the bread-maker, and tried out a healthy dessert recipe from my quitting sugar book.

It was so good to see them! I was nervous; it was the first time I'd had any of the Loose Women round to my house, and I wanted them to like it. It seems crazy, but we tend to meet up in London because we live all over the place, so I was really flattered that they were making the effort to come out to Surrey to see me.

The afternoon raced by as we caught up on our latest news and gossip. Mum and Dad came round too, and we all sat outside on the porch in the October sunshine. It couldn't have gone any better, even though my dessert was a disaster – even lovely Linda said it was the most disgusting thing she'd ever had! I was happily exhausted when they left.

Day 13

My forty-seventh birthday. I didn't feel right when I woke up – just 'out of sorts', and I'd had a sweaty, uncomfortable night. It was my birthday, though, and I knew the kids and Nick would have something planned for me. I went downstairs and sure enough, I heard hissed voices: 'She's coming! She's coming!' As I walked into the kitchen, I saw it was covered with birthday banners and a clutch of bright, helium-filled balloons.

'Happy Birthday, Mum!'

Amy had made a little film for me on her phone: a montage of photos of us together, with a song called 'My Mum'. I was in bits by the end of it. Nick had gone shopping with all the kids to get me things, and between them they'd chosen some lovely clothes that I needed while I was recovering. New leggings for wearing round the house; a lovely top and a fluffy jumper; a huge, soft, cosy scarf – I was touched by their thoughtfulness.

The kids headed off to school and I got dressed.
I felt as if I was wading through treacle, I was so tired.
A delivery van arrived to drop off two gleaming,
rose gold-coloured martini glasses from Sally, my editor
at *Loose Women*. She's known for her love of Vespers, a
lethal cocktail served in these glasses, and we'd pledged
to go out for another 'Vesper session' when I was better.
I propped them up in the box and left them in my
bedroom so I could see them.

Nick and I then headed to Esher for a wander round
the shops and lunch before he headed off to see his girls
in Eastbourne, as he does every Wednesday. I felt queasy
as I sipped my favourite drink – a Kir royale – which he'd
thoughtfully ordered for me, and ate as much of my meal
as I could manage.

Once home, I went to bed as soon as Nick left, and
slept for the rest of the afternoon, waking up just before
my parents arrived with cake and presents. It's a tradition
that we always have family birthdays at my house, and
they're normally loud, fun, jolly affairs, with all of us
crammed into the kitchen, music playing, lots of food,
and Jackson barking as we sing 'Happy Birthday'. I love it,
and wouldn't have it any other way.

Today though, I couldn't stand for long so I sat in an
armchair like a nana. Mum had made and brought with
her a curry – to save me cooking – so I watched as she set
everything up. We had a quiet few hours as the kids went
about their normal daily routine of after-school clubs and
dog walking, then we ate, had cake, and played a random
game of 'guess which wild animals come from which
country', devised by Amy and which seemed to last for an

eternity. I barely moved, and even Dad nodded off on the sofa. It was very far removed from a normal birthday, and I hoped I hadn't spoiled it for everyone by being quiet.

I put the kids to bed and was heading up myself when Nick got home. The following day was going to be busy for him, making up for taking a full day off, and he had an early start planned before travelling to Birmingham, so he came up too.

As soon as my head hit the pillow I knew it was going to be a rough night. I just couldn't settle. I was so tired – exhausted even – but my mind was racing and my body was twitching with tension. I wasn't able to keep my arms and legs still, and I knew I was disturbing Nick. Rolling over was still tricky – I had to think and brace myself before I moved, and I couldn't get comfortable.

Two hours later I gave up and went to the spare room. I watched TV on my iPad until almost 2 a.m., then dozed until 3.30, got up and went to the loo, then tried to settle myself. My pillow was soaked with sour sweat, and I couldn't shake the feeling of restlessness. I must have nodded off eventually because I woke up to the kids getting ready for school. I came downstairs to make sure everyone was OK, which they were because, as ever, wonderful Lin was there.

Day 14

Thank God for Lin. She ensured life carried on as normal, so the kids kept their routine and the house ran like clockwork. Lin has worked for me since Amy was six months old and I was juggling two jobs – *GMTV* and *Loose Women*. I was permanently exhausted from getting up at 3.30 a.m. every day, being sent all over the country at a moment's notice, heading back to London to host *Loose Women*, and then home to my young family.

Over the past ten years Lin has become much more than someone who helps me with childcare; she's become my 'other mum' and my right-hand woman. She keeps my home life steady and is part of our family. She was my rock when I was getting divorced and became ill with stress and worry, and she was my champion when things turned a corner and began to right themselves. Lin keeps our little ship steady and, if I'm honest, she looks after me as much as she does Amy and Fin.

I waved everyone off and wobbled back to bed. I felt dreadful – exhausted, queasy and smelly from my horrible night. I felt anxious, too. Was this normal? To feel so wiped out after feeling OK? I could only think that I must have pushed myself too hard when Linda and Nadia came round – but I'd enjoyed it!

I wasn't in as much pain now, apart from the odd internal 'twang' if I stretched too hard or moved too quickly. I'd taken things easy, and only done what I felt capable of at the time. Maybe my brain was further along than my body, and now they were even – they both felt like mush.

Things didn't really improve until much later in the day after I'd watched *Loose Women*, *Judge Rinder* and *Who's Doing the Dishes?*. I barely moved from my chair until the kids came back from school and I realized Nick would be home soon too. So I had a shower and dressed in my daytime pyjama uniform of baggy bottoms and a sweatshirt. Nick was exhausted when he got back from work, so we got an early night in.

Day 15

It was Nick's turn to have a restless night and he gave up at 3 a.m. and headed downstairs. It's like Piccadilly Circus round here at night these days! I'd taken two Kalms Night tablets and spritzed some of the pillow spray Linda Robson had given me and, thank God, I made it through until 7 a.m. A good night's sleep at last.

I got up to see if the kids and Nick were OK, and they were all downstairs getting ready for the day. Lin was in, ready to take Amy to school. I was standing next to her, talking through a play date that Amy was going on after school and sorting out the following week, when Jackson pushed past me to sniff at the floor. I glanced down and was mortified: I was leaking. Big blobs of dark brown blood were splattered on the kitchen floor, and the dog was licking them up.

I didn't know whether to be horrified or relieved, as I wasn't sure if Lin had noticed. If she had, she was very kind and didn't mention anything. I gave Amy a hug and felt another trickle down my leg as I smiled and waved her off from the doorstep. As soon as the front door closed, I grabbed a wad of tissues and shoved them between my legs before stumbling upstairs. I thought I'd finished with this, but obviously not. Maybe it was because I'd been lying down for so long, and then stood up? I had a shower, then put a bigger sanitary pad in my knickers, rather than the panty liners I'd been using just in case. It wasn't fresh blood that was leaking out of me – it looked like old, stale blood from the surgery. I'd been told this would happen so I wasn't necessarily worried, but it did feel odd that it had been in me all this time.

I felt down, with a niggling and building anxiety. It was like that feeling you get when there's an exam coming up and you haven't studied. Or when you're waiting for some news, and you're convinced it's going to be bad. All day I had a knot in my stomach and my head felt strange. I tried to reason with myself that it was all normal. That my hormones were always going to take time to settle down, and the ride was always going to be a little bit bumpy.

I had an email yesterday about returning to work on *Loose Women*, and my dates have been changed from one day at the start of the week and one day at the end, to three days on the trot. I'm quietly panicking that I won't be able to do it. Not three days in a row without a breathing space in the middle to recover. I'm nervous about telling them that I don't think I'm ready. I still feel exhausted following a visit from friends; how on earth can I cope with *work*?

The worry buzzed around my head all day. I'm terrible at saying no, but I really don't feel that in two weeks' time I'll be ready to hit the ground running and be the sparkling, capable self they need me to be. I also have four different charity events lined up for my second week back, that I've promised I'll attend. I don't want to let anyone down but I'm growing anxious at the thought of being there and having to stand for all that time, smiling and laughing and being 'on'. As things stand, I get tired just listening to the kids talk about their day – how can I go to work, then to another event in the evening, for four nights in a row?

By late afternoon, things had gone round and round my head to the point where I felt sick, so I emailed Sally, the *Loose Women* editor, told her how I was feeling, and that I thought I should take the full six weeks off rather than four. Within an hour I got an email back, telling me not to get stressed about it; they would find a way round it, and to take as much time as I needed. Relief surged through me. I had more time.

Day 16

Nick and I *both* managed to get a full night's sleep, which was fantastic. I made everyone pancakes for breakfast, as Saturday is always pancake day, then Nick and the children got ready and headed off to Eastbourne. I stayed behind on my own – I still didn't feel up to a long drive and socializing all day. I knew it would wipe me out and I still wasn't quite feeling myself, which meant there was a good chance I'd get tired and grumpy with all the kids' noise, which wasn't fair on anyone.

That night in bed, I was lying on my back, waiting for Nick to finish getting ready, and I rolled over to turn off my bedside light. I did it without thinking, or bracing myself, and oh my God, something inside went *twang*. Pain shot through me and my body went into spasm. My abdomen seized up. I couldn't move. Nick rushed round to my side of the bed and stood over me, concern all over his lovely face.

'What did you do? Are you OK? What can I do?'

I lay on my side with my eyes squeezed shut and told him what had happened. He helped me roll gently on to my back again and pulled the duvet up to my chin, tucking me in like a child and turning out the light. My muscles were still clamped tightly in a painful spasm around whichever part of me it was that had pulled, and I lay still, trying to breathe the tension out of my body. I lay in the dark for an eternity, long after Nick had checked again that I was OK and had fallen asleep himself, with one hand resting on me reassuringly. I panicked that I'd ruptured internal stitches and mentally kicked myself for being so stupid. Having the operation was one thing, dealing with the aftermath was the difficult part – and I'd only just begun.

Day 17

The next morning, the pain had eased. Sleep had come eventually and had been the best thing for it, as I obviously relaxed and so too did the spasm. I'd definitely damaged something, though, because I had a dull ache all day. I was still leaking dark brown blood; I could feel it coming out of me as I stood chatting to my parents' friends that afternoon, and as I helped Mum get canapés out of the oven. It wasn't fresh blood though, so I knew I hadn't ruptured anything, or burst some stitches.

That day was my parents' fiftieth wedding anniversary drinks at their house. It was actually the second party they'd held to mark the occasion; the first had been in Scotland on their actual anniversary a few weeks ago. This one was for their friends rather than the Scottish clan.

I made a real effort and got dressed up for the first time since my operation. It took for ever. I even clipped in some hair pieces to thicken my horribly thin hair. It had been bad before the operation, but now it seemed to have lost the will to live. It was limp, lank and receding around my hairline. None of this was particularly new, but now my extensions were out, I could really see it. I'd had them removed to give my hair a break while I was recovering, and as anyone who usually wears extensions will know, it's a shock to go back to your normal, fine, thin hair after having had a headful!

I put on some sparkly jewellery – my feather ring and some funky earrings – the lovely top that the kids had chosen for my birthday, tight black trousers and black heels. I could pull the trousers up easily because of the weight I'd lost, but buttoning them was a different story. My stomach was still swollen, and the waistband rubbed against my scars.

I didn't want to wear leggings any more, though; I wanted to dress nicely, so I left the trousers unbuttoned and used a black hairband to fasten them. I looped it round the button, threaded it through the buttonhole, twisted it to make another small loop, then pulled it back over the button again. I tugged the waistband down below my scars, pulled my top over the trousers and ta-da! No one would know. I was knackered by the time I'd finished getting ready – goodness knows where I was going to find the energy to leave the house and socialize – but it was nice to look in the mirror and see *me*.

Day 18

I woke up with Nick at 5.30 a.m. as he had his fortnightly early start to take the girls back to Eastbourne. I lay in bed until 7, then got up to see to my two. Amy was being a bit of a smart alec, acting cheeky and answering back, so I needed to nip that in the bud. I had a feeling that iPad confiscation was on the cards.

I felt good today. I think I was so relieved that I had more time to get better before going back to work that it was as if a weight had been lifted. And a cloud. I was doing so much better in myself. I meditated for the first time in a week, and then felt like a fool for not having done it at the very time when I needed it most – when I was feeling cloudy and low. Still, I was back on track again.

I made an effort getting dressed again, and for the second day in a row I didn't just put on my comfy leggings and a jumper or sweatshirt. OK, I still wore leggings, but I actually wore a bra – and that's a *big deal* at home. I don't bother unless I'm out of the house, bloody uncomfortable things. And a nice wrap dress/jumper and a swishy cardigan thing. Even though I knew I was going to be alone in the house all day, I did it for me.

I was still leaking. It felt like the blood from the surgery was all coming out now. I hoped it was normal. It wasn't fresh, so I wasn't too worried about it, but I couldn't help wondering where it had been all this time – why had it taken so long to leave my body? I'd googled 'discharge after hysterectomy' and knew that it was normal, but I couldn't help but think. It was another reason why I wanted to try to look nice on the outside at least, because it felt pretty disgusting knowing what was going on underneath the layers . . .

I picked the scabs off my scars today, and managed to gently wipe the remnants of the plasters off my skin with baby oil and a cotton pad. Even that made me feel better.

My Lara Croft bullet wounds aren't as noticeable now, just four neat little scars dotted across my battlefield of a stomach. That's what Nick and I have been calling them, anyway, which makes us both laugh, and me feel like an action hero rather than a middle-aged woman. To be fair, I don't think an action hero could go through this – I'd like to see Superman fight off baddies with half his insides removed, emotions all over the place and that thick slick of dark hair he runs his fingers through reduced to a few pathetic strands. Kryptonite has nothing on a hysterectomy, Mr Man of Steel. It's about time Menopause Woman joined the ranks of the Justice League – that'd have the alien invaders scampering back to their planet in a hot flush!

Day 19

My alarm went off at 7 a.m. after another full night's sleep – hurrah! I've been taking the Kalms Night every night, which I hope is OK, but it's working so I'm going to stick with it for now. Nick and I meditated before getting up with the kids – I've decided we're going to fit it in every day, and this is the only way to make sure it gets done. It doesn't take long and makes a huge difference, for both of us.

I felt calm today, and still. My brain switched into meditation mode easily because I'd done it yesterday, and I only mentally beat myself up for a moment for not doing it last week, because at least I was back at it again. Just ten minutes and I felt ready to deal with the day.

I'm leaking like crazy now – dark brown liquid. I've googled it – yes, again – and apparently it is normal to have brown discharge for 4–6 weeks after a hysterectomy as the internal wounds heal. I've also noticed my glands under my left arm are enlarged and the area is tender, which I'm assuming is just my body sorting itself out. I don't feel unwell, so I'm sure it's OK. It is OK, isn't it?!

I've decided to book an appointment with Dr Tina Peers. I haven't seen her for a couple of years. Now I've most definitely leapt off the menopausal cliff, it would be a good idea to get her opinion on the best way to transform my leap into an uplifting flight rather than an epic faceplant.

Day 21

A quiet day, when I never quite felt myself. Lots of ringing round trying to get an appointment with Dr Peers. It's the first thing I've had to do for myself that involves the outside world, and I barely know what day it is. How on earth are menopausal women, who can't even get to the top of the stairs without forgetting what they've gone up there for, expected to handle booking an appointment?

Day 22

I had a lovely few hours with Donna, the make-up artist friend who set me up on a blind date with Nick three years ago. She arrived with fresh flowers, magazines, a small embroidery kit, a cool bag with ingredients for lunch, fresh turmeric (which is good for healing) to grate into meals and drinks, and a bottle of arnica oil (good for bruising). Oh, and sugar- and dairy-free chocolate so I can have a treat but stick to my low-sugar regime. She laughed when I told her wine was back on the menu again, even if biscuits aren't . . .

I finally managed to get through to another clinic where Dr Peers works. It's further away, but at least I managed to speak to someone, and booked an appointment for next week. I'm looking forward to speaking to someone who specializes in menopause management and to make sure I'm on the right track.

I'd also like to get some blood tests to check my hormone levels; the testosterone gel I've been given to apply has brought me out in spots of adolescent proportions. They are *huge*. Angry red lumps and pustules are dappled across my neck, shoulders and back. This is not the look I want. I know that testosterone is good for my energy levels and my libido (which is now nestling at a few bars above flatline), but there has to be some other way that doesn't leave me looking like I'm going through my plooky youth all over again – it was bad enough the first time.

A month after my operation I finally saw Dr Peers, who was exactly as I hoped she'd be: professional, helpful and still as passionate as ever about women's sexual and reproductive health. She agreed that I should get my blood tested to see where my hormone levels were. She also recommended that I come off the testosterone for a few weeks to let my levels settle down, then introduce it again, but more slowly this time. She also prescribed me progesterone tablets to help keep any remaining endometriosis at bay (it hadn't occurred to me that it wasn't all gone but, as she pointed out, short of opening up my whole body there was no way of knowing for sure) and oestrogen pessaries to help keep things elasticated internally.

Dr Peers knows how important it is to feel good about yourself; that having a hysterectomy shouldn't mean the end of your life physically, emotionally and sexually. I was only forty-seven – I wasn't dead yet! It's a crime that she and doctors like her aren't available around the country on the NHS. She's not seen as a necessary service. Surely making sure that *millions* of women are carrying on their lives as healthy, functioning human beings, keeping strong, mentally and physically, and contributing to their families and society until a ripe old age is important!

It makes me *rage* to think that the menopause is swept aside as 'women's problems'; that we are supposed to just live with the symptoms which so many men roll their eyes at and ignore. Just because in the past women's health has been treated as something we deal with stoically until we keel over, doesn't mean it has to carry on this way. Surely it would *save* the NHS money each year if we made sure that women are as fit and well as they can be, so that we can carry on being wives, mothers, sisters, grandmothers, friends, employers and employees, and carrying the responsibilities that those roles bring – namely helping everyone else!

I also went to see my GP to make sure that my prescription was clear, so that when the time came for it to be picked up at my local chemist, nothing would be missing. I wanted to talk to her about my problems sleeping, too – after a spell of getting into a pattern of 'all right' sleep, every night had become a drama of lying in bed for hours, getting more and more agitated and stressed about the fact that my body was twitching with tiredness and my eyes were heavy, but for the life of me I couldn't get them both to switch off so that I could go to sleep.

My head was full of bees, buzzing with useless, stressful thoughts that even my usual mindfulness techniques couldn't quiet. Just as I started to relax, my leg would cramp, or my arm, and I'd have to move just to ease the pain, which jolted me out of my deep breathing. On top of that there was Nick's snoring!

My GP was awesome. She listened and agreed that I needed help; that it's difficult enough to recover from a major operation such as a hysterectomy, without throwing in insomnia as well. She prescribed me some non-addictive sleeping tablets and told me to take them for five nights on the trot to break the cycle of getting stressed about sleeping.

The first night I tried them . . . oh my word. It was heaven. I woke up nine hours later with no recollection of even having nodded off. Nick had got up, showered, dressed and was downstairs helping the kids get ready, and I hadn't heard a *thing*. Wow. It was weird, but brilliant.

By the fifth week following the operation, I was still having good and bad days. I did a Christmas photoshoot for work and it took me days to recover from it. I was exhausted by the time I got home, and I hadn't had to do anything other than socialize and have my picture taken by a lovely photographer and a team of people I really enjoyed working with. Nadia, Kaye and Coleen were there, and it was great to see them and catch up, but they seemed so vibrant and strong compared to me. Was I ever that energetic, I wondered? Would I ever be again?

That week was also Hallowe'en and we invited some neighbours over. There are so many families with little tots in our close and I love to have them round to trick-or-treat. It was a really nice evening but yet again, despite being absolutely wiped out with the effort of socializing, I couldn't sleep. When I did, I had stressful, restless dreams and woke up drenched in sweat, my hair stuck to my head.

Kicking the duvet off made me cold, having it on made me hot. I wanted to sob with the frustration of it all. Then my internal scars started to throb, but I couldn't be bothered to get up to take some painkillers, so I lay in the dark, willing myself to sleep so I wouldn't feel the discomfort any more.

Eventually I gave in, though, and went to the bathroom for some paracetamol and some Kalms, and tried again. I didn't want to take the sleeping tablets as it felt too late in the night, and I didn't want to be woozy the next day. Luckily, the Kalms worked, and the next thing I knew it was morning and my alarm was ringing me out of my deepest sleep of the night. Oh, the bloody injustice.

I was stressed all day about not getting enough sleep for work when the time came to go back, and about being too tired to function properly. When would I feel better? Was I rushing things, or should I be further along by now? I looked at the hysterectomy website that Kaye Adams had recommended to me, and I wished I hadn't. I became convinced that I'd done everything wrong and was going to feel this dreadful for months and months. I thought I'd sat down too long when I should have been moving around. I worried that I'd done too *much* moving around when I should have been sitting down. I beat myself up for drinking wine in the evening, for walking to the shops, for trying to feel 'normal'. In theory I'd done nothing wrong, but my anxious brain was having none of it.

By Week 6 it was time to return to work! I was so scared the night before that I took a sleeping tablet and actually managed to get a full night – thank God. I was nervous – the-first-day-back-at-school-after-the-summer-holidays kind of nervous, when you worry that your friends won't want to speak to you any more because they've moved on, and you won't know what the teacher is talking about, or remember how to string a sentence together.

Physically, although I could get up and dressed, and walk about, I still got tired very, very quickly. Adrenaline carried me through my journey to work, commuting into London on the train in the dark, stopping to buy some breakfast and snacks for the day, then walking from the station to the studio.

The morning meeting was a joyous reunion, and the show itself was warm and lovely. I couldn't have hoped for better. I had an overwhelming response from the audience, which was wonderful, but what was truly amazing that day was the reaction of the team. I've worked in telly for over twenty years and have taken time off twice, to have my babies. Each time I returned to work after twelve weeks, and each time it was a case of, 'Oh, you're back', and I'd get straight back to it, taking care not to whinge. This time I could feel the warmth and love from the team, though, who were genuinely pleased that I was there.

On my way home, the adrenaline began to wear off and the tiredness crept back in. It seeped into my whole body, through my skin and into my bones, so that by the time I got to my front door, I was mentally and physically exhausted. I wiped off all the beautifully applied make-up, dragged my expertly coiffed hair back into a ponytail, pulled on comfy clothes that didn't sit on my scars, and collapsed in front of the telly with the kids until bedtime.

My second day back was a big one for the show – not because of me, but because it was dedicated to Robbie Williams and his lovely wife and fellow Loose Woman, Ayda. It was a great day. They were both so nervous when we started filming, but then I saw their shoulders drop, they breathed out, and they re-lax-ed.

Robbie was himself, not the performer or showman that you see on late-night chat shows. He was there as a husband and a dad – just a guy talking about his life, his feelings, his experiences. I loved making him and Ayda feel comfortable enough to be themselves, and I felt well enough to be able to help make that happen. Ayda was apprehensive because her husband was in her domain, and she wanted to protect him but also do her job. However, her body language relaxed when she saw he was OK, and she sat back and let him do his thing. It was one of my proudest days, though it did take it out of me.

That evening was an awards do – the Mind Media Awards. Knowing how tired I was, the runners at the *Loose Women* studio were amazing and found me a spare dressing room to stay in for the afternoon so that I could get some rest. I lay on the sofa, covered myself with my coat and slept for a few hours. When my alarm pinged, I dragged myself up, wiped my smudged eye make-up from under my eyes with my fingers and went out to meet Nadia, editor Sally and Siobhan, our deputy editor, to head to the awards.

The show had been nominated for our 'Lighten the Load' campaign, which we'd launched earlier in the year and had talked about a lot. Encouraging viewers to open up about their own problems – and get help – felt like the right thing for the show to do, especially because we ourselves had been so open on the programme about our own issues.

Our campaign had launched with me speaking honestly and nervously about my experience of postnatal depression. I'd written about it before, but actually saying things out loud on camera had been very different. And difficult.

That night we were in an incredible category, up against Grayson Perry talking about the difficulties of being a man, *The Island with Bear Grylls*, and Prince Harry's *DIY SOS* special on veterans with post-traumatic stress. When the clips of the nominated shows played on screen, I felt a jolt when my own face filled the room. I'd not watched the footage of myself talking and hadn't realized how nervous I'd sounded, and hesitant. I'd rushed through what I had to say; my words clear but running into one another as I choked my way through my deeply personal story.

In the theatre, my face grew hot and prickly, and before I knew it, tears were running down my cheeks as I watched the gigantic screen and the woman who was somehow holding it together while talking about how broken she felt. That was *me*. It was me then and, what nobody realized, it was me still, despite all the physical changes I was going through. I was still me.

'And the winner is . . . *Loose Women* for their "Lighten the Load" campaign!'

Nadia and I looked at each other and screamed – we'd won! The four of us gathered ourselves together and made our way to the stage, applause ringing in our ears. Sally gave a speech, talking about how we'd been inspired to launch the campaign following the tragic suicide of our colleague June Sarpong's brother. It was a terrible thing that we had spoken about candidly, in a way that only *Loose Women* can, and it had opened the floodgates for us to talk about other mental-health issues that had affected us personally.

Nadia spoke next about the power of oversharing and talking to your friends, as we do on the show. Then, I took the mic and admitted that I'd just cried watching myself on screen, because I'd never seen the clip before. I said that one of the things *Loose Women* did so well was to take huge issues, such as suicide or depression, and make them small and personal. Because when those things are happening to you, you feel as if you're the only one to feel that way.

Watching the clip had made me realize that if I was sat at home struggling, I'd be so thankful to know that someone who might look as if they had their life together was telling me they felt the same way I did. But, I said, don't do what I did and wait until it's over before talking about it. Speak up and get help when you need it, because there's no need to suffer for longer. I finished by saying that I was so proud of *Loose Women* and the campaign, and hoped it was just the start of something.

I made a decision that night to take my own advice. The next time I felt down or in pain, I was going to say something and do something about it right away, not hope it would go away by itself . . . because it won't. It will just grow and grow until it's so big and slippery that you can't handle it on your own.

That's why we need to 'confess' to how we're feeling, because it's the only way we can hope to do anything about it. Whether it's speaking to a doctor or opening up to a trusted friend, talking is the first of many steps towards feeling less frightened of whatever it is we're going through. The menopause can be an incredibly isolating experience, as the body that you've come to know throughout your adult life changes beyond your recognition and understanding, and not many of those changes are positive ones.

I know, from my experience, and from those of the women who have reached out to me, that losing your sense of self is one of the most dominant factors in making women feel alone during this time. I can't stress this to you strongly enough – you are *not alone*. We are all with you, and we are all in this together. We've got this.

Dr Peers Says . . .

HYSTERECTOMIES – THE INS AND OUTS, SO TO SPEAK . . .

A hysterectomy is the surgical removal of the uterus (womb). It's a very common operation – one in five women in the UK undergo a hysterectomy before they reach the age of fifty-five. Reasons for a hysterectomy include endometriosis; painful, heavy or frequent periods that have not responded to medical treatment; fibroids (swellings of abnormal muscle in the womb) that cause bleeding and pain; uterine prolapse; and gynaecological cancer.

There are different types of hysterectomy. The most common is a total abdominal hysterectomy where both the body and neck of the womb are removed, including the fallopian tubes and ovaries. The alternative is a subtotal hysterectomy, where only the womb is removed. In the case of the latter, women will still have a cervix and should continue to have cervical smears.

Once you've had a hysterectomy, you no longer have periods and you can't get pregnant. If you have your ovaries removed during surgery, it's likely that you'll experience the menopause earlier than expected. It's extremely important to consider HRT after removal of the ovaries, especially if the woman is under the age of fifty.[1]

THE POTENTIAL MENTAL FALLOUT

Many women experience a huge sense of relief after a hysterectomy as often they feel much better and finally pain-free (as in the case of endometriosis) for the first time in many years.

However, there may also be a sense of loss. Removal of your womb and the inability to conceive a child can affect how you feel as a woman and your desire to have sex. The psychological effects of a hysterectomy can be difficult for your partner to understand and you may also have difficulty discussing how you feel with friends or family. It's important that you talk to someone and seek help and support where you can.[2]

TREATMENTS THEN AND NOW

Although hysterectomy is still a common procedure, it's performed much less often than it used to be. Over the years, the womb (and the fallopian tubes, ovaries, cervix and parts of the vagina) have been removed for all sorts of gynaecological reasons – from hysteria to abnormal bleeding. These days, the decision to have a hysterectomy is not taken quite so lightly.

The majority of hysterectomies are performed for conditions such as fibroids, endometriosis, and uterine prolapse, where other medical options have been tried and failed. However, newer treatment approaches for fibroids and heavy menstrual bleeding are replacing the need for a hysterectomy for many women. For example, high-frequency ultrasound or minimally invasive surgery is being used to shrink or remove fibroids, and intrauterine devices containing the hormone progesterone can reduce endometrial wall thickening and control excessive menstrual bleeding. For those women with severe uterine prolapse or large fibroids, a hysterectomy may be the only option to relieve symptoms. However, even then, the pros and cons of undergoing surgery must always be carefully considered.[3]

RECOVERING FROM A HYSTERECTOMY: DOS AND DON'TS

Hysterectomy is a major surgical procedure and the time to full recovery varies from woman to woman. In general, you should expect to walk briefly the day after surgery and then exercise gently, under instruction from a physiotherapist, within a few days. Keeping moving after surgery is important to maintain good circulation and reduce the risk of blood clots. Activities such as swimming, driving and sexual intercourse can resume after about six weeks, providing all is well at the post-operative check. You can also think about returning to work as long as your job doesn't involve heavy lifting.

As your body adjusts, you'll experience a number of sensations that are normal and should not cause concern. These include slight vaginal bleeding or brown discharge, trapped wind and indigestion due to lack of movement, constipation and backache, and discomfort or 'pinging sensations' in the abdomen. Signs that all is not well and you should return to your doctor include the presence of additional pain, pus, fresh blood or smelly discharge, or feeling faint or hot and feverish.

1 Sources: WHC. Hysterectomy Fact Sheet. www.womens-health-concern. org; The Hysterectomy Association. Fact Sheet – What is a Hysterectomy? www.hysterectomy-association.org.uk

2 Source: WHC. Hysterectomy Fact Sheet. www.womens-health-concern.org

3 Source: From Dr Oz: www.doctoroz.com/article/1-surgery-women-dont-need-hysterectomy

4

Let's Talk about Sex

'I'm a healthy person, happily married, but my sex drive is zero. My poor husband! He's amazing and so very tolerant. A real gent . . . I guess what he has done is "given up" . . . I feel so awful but I can't get things going!'

'We've had no sex life for about five to six years. Can't bear the thought of it. Just no interest on my part.'

'When I first began the menopause, I was not interested in sex at all – would kiss and cuddle but that was it. But in the last year I've completely turned around and, not wanting to be rude, I cannot get enough. I'm not complaining, though.'

Sex. There, I've said it. OK, I've whispered it. *S-e-e-e-e-e-x-x-x-x-x* . . . Sex, sex, sex, sex, sex . . . It's such a strange word when you write it down, or say it out loud, or even think about it. 'It', as we casually refer to that most intimate of activities, doesn't really feature in the day-to-day conversations of middle-aged women dropping their kids at school, walking

95

the dog or rushing off to work. But we all do it. Some more than others, and some hardly at all, but either way it plays a *huge* part in our lives.

We worried about it in our teens, had fun with it in our twenties, focused on the practicalities of it in our thirties, fretted about the possible lack of outcome from it in our forties, wondered if we'd ever feel the same way about it again in our fifties, and decided we *wouldn't* feel the same way about it ever again from our sixties – and that was OK!

Whatever your experience of sex has been throughout your life – good, bad or indifferent – the menopause is one of those times when it most definitely changes. If you've had children, then it's right up there with post-baby sex – you either get right back in the saddle (if you know what I mean) and barely miss a beat; or you grit your teeth and bear it while internally raging that this is *yet another* thing you have to do. Or you decide that horse riding was never really your thing and you'd rather poke yourself in the eye with a sharp stick than let anyone or anything get in the way of sleep/work/ friends/wine/box sets/more sleep . . .

I think how you feel comes down to two factors – body and mind – and the two are inextricably linked. Our body changes during the menopause; that goes without saying. It just doesn't seem to work the way it used to. The parts of you that were normally dry are now soaked (think upper lip, back of neck) and the parts that you relied on to get wet when needed are now bone dry (you *know* where I mean). How's that for luck?

All of this leaves you feeling rubbish about yourself, which then starts to play havoc with your mind . . . How are you supposed to feel sexy when your body is falling apart, everything is the wrong way around, you have no energy, your brain has turned to mush, your libido has dropped through the floor, and everything your partner says and does makes you want to punch him on the nose?

Feeling bad about sex is awful, and all the evening prim-rose oil and deep breathing exercises in the world aren't going to get you over this one. It's something we hear about often, and something most of us enjoy having a good-natured (and occasionally not-so-good-natured) grumble about, talking round the edges of it, but never actually getting down to the nitty-gritty. Why is that?

No sex, please, we're British

How much sex is too much sex? How infrequently is too little? You can't move for sex being thrust in your face in adverts, movies, TV dramas, books, magazine articles, newspaper headlines ... Everybody is either at it, or wanting to be. It's interesting to note that once you start paying attention, most of these people wriggling and writhing about are in their thir-ties or younger, and fit neatly into the slim, golden-skinned and flicky-haired bracket of improbable women. And men, for that matter. You don't see many who are struggling with middle-aged spread, sweaty foreheads and a libido that has crawled away to die somewhere.

Once a woman reaches a certain age (which the media has decided is somewhere just beyond puberty, apparently), she's no longer seen as a sexual being. Of course there are exceptions. I for one thought that Gillian Anderson was rather marvellous in the BBC drama *The Fall* (that's the one where everyone fancied Jamie Dornan, even though he played a psy-chopathic serial killer). Most 'women of a certain age' who are portrayed as having a keen sexual appetite are also seen as having some kind of flaw: they're either damaged, selfish and arrogant, a tart with a heart, or just a downright slapper. Why isn't it OK for an older woman to have a healthy sexual appetite?

During my online conversation with women through social media, countless individuals opened up to me about many aspects of their menopause and were more than happy to talk about how they felt going into it – problems they'd experienced in the build-up and as it became full-blown, and what they found to be useful when it came to dealing with the many symptoms. What they *didn't* want to talk about, however, was sex.

The quotes at the beginning of this chapter were some of the responses I got from brave and delightful women who were open to discussing how the menopause had affected their sex drive, but in comparison to other symptoms, which got a lot of coverage, the replies about sex were much less forthcoming. It was interesting, however, that the responses I got were split between women who were at completely opposite ends of the scale. Sex was either a complete no-no, or a resounding yes-yes-yes! There was very little in between.

Of the women who got in touch with me to say that sex was off the agenda, all of them felt as if their libido had just disappeared once they entered the menopause. One woman put it beautifully:

'I've no interest in it any more! I'm forty-six and postmenopausal . . . been on HRT since Feb 2017 . . . My husband is very understanding and doesn't pester me but I do feel bad, and at bedtime I dread him touching me! I hope it will get better soon. I clam up if I think sex is on the cards.'

On the other hand, another woman summed up how sex had entered a different phase during the menopause, and one she was very happy with:

> *'On HRT for four years. Married for thirty-four. Have*
> *fab, amazing sex with my hubby . . . Gets better and better!*
> *It's all about communication, I think.'*

I think she's on to something: we just don't talk about sex, either as couples or otherwise. Now, I don't believe that's because women aren't interested in it. I just think that as Brits we don't like to talk about the subject. It's right up there with how much money we earn, or whether someone has BO. You just don't bring it up in conversation. It's such a shame because sex, whether it's the lack of it or otherwise, is an important part of the menopause journey.

So, I'm going to take a deep breath and talk about it, because I know that there are menopausal women out there who are interested to know whether their sex life is 'normal' and, if they aren't happy, what they can do about it.

Loose talk

I work with some incredible ladies on *Loose Women*, and the discussions we have off air are far more revealing than the ones that are broadcast to the nation. That's because we can be truly open and honest without worrying what anyone thinks about us. We're friends as well as colleagues and we don't judge, no matter how dramatic the confession. We say what we *really* feel without having to edit ourselves. And yes, we talk about sex. It is, however, the one subject that we joke and skirt around, as none of us likes to admit that whatever is happening – or not happening – between the sheets at home could be a problem.

Ninety-nine per cent of the time the conversation revolves around 'duty sex', or how often having sex is something done to keep the peace. Strategies are discussed:

'Do it as soon as you get there when you go on holiday! That way he won't feel hard done by when you keep putting him off!'

'Get him drunk and then tell him you did have sex last night, he just can't remember!'

'I say I've got my period again, even though that's now three times this month . . . !'

'I put on an Oscar-winning performance last night, even though I was doing my Sainsbury's shopping in my head . . .'

'I just let him get on with it, at least I don't have to think about it for another few weeks – tick!'

These comments are so commonplace that we don't even think about how strange – and awful – they are. The fact is that not one of those jokey comments involves us doing something that makes us feel good. Is this because we've been somehow programmed to think that enjoying sex, and being open about what we want and how we feel, is selfish? Is it something that only self-absorbed women do, the kind of women who don't put their husband and children first, but think about what *they* want?

Or is it because some women feel that nothing gets done the way they like it if they aren't in charge or across it all domestically – that's a fact in many (not all, but many) busy, chaotic family homes – so making time and energy for sex is difficult to say the least. Quite frankly, those of us in the 'sandwich generation' – balancing children's needs with those of ageing parents – have enough stress to deal with without factoring in feeling sexy and attractive. And a lot of the time, these stresses come to the fore just when your menopause sets in. So it's hardly surprising that thinking about sex – never mind actually enjoying it – is right at the bottom of your to-do list.

Not wanting sex at all is extremely common during the menopause and can, of course, have nothing to do with the external pressures of family or work. The decline or loss of libido can have various physiological causes, with the tailing off of certain hormones being right at the top of the list.

I think our attitude to sex is a product of a mixture of these things, both physical and mental, and it's complex. So this is where communication comes in again. It's good to talk. Talk to someone. Confess, if you like . . . Share the load, whether it's to release emotionally so that you don't feel so pent-up and filled with repressed fury that *you're* always the one rushing round sorting *everything* out, or to find a way to get the practical support you need so that you're not doing it all by yourself. Not talking means no change, and if you're happy with that, then fine. But if you aren't, then you need to do something about it.

Not wanting sex is OK. I really want to stress that. There's no right or wrong when it comes to your libido – it's whatever you're happy and comfortable with, and what works within the dynamics of your relationship. If both of you are content as you are, then that's wonderful and long may it continue.

Problems can creep in when one of you *isn't* happy with the sexual set-up. Feeling put-upon is never a good thing. In our day-to-day lives we can often feel like the commander of a busy ship, with everyone wanting a piece of us and expecting us to sort things out so that *their* lives run smoothly, but here I mean put-upon in the bedroom. That doing-it-just-to-keep-the-ship-afloat kind of sex. Nobody likes that; not you and, if you asked, probably not him either. He wants your heart to be in it, and your head.

So what can you do?

Step one. If you want to do something about it, have a think about what has changed for you. Is it simply exhaustion from carrying too much of the load at home? If it is, then talk about it with your family, and see if daily chores can be spread out a bit. You don't get a medal when you're dead for having done more ironing than the person lying in the ground next to you, or for being the only one to have walked the dog or done the school run. Try to find a way to lighten your load.

Step two. How are you feeling? Has the fire literally gone out? Do you *never* feel like it any more? If you genuinely don't feel like ever having sex again, and this is a far cry from how you used to feel about it, how does that make you feel? Not bothered? Sad? Angry? Once you've got it clear in your own head and you have some kind of idea about what – if anything – you'd like to do about it, *talk to your partner*.

This isn't something you can sort out on your own. Open a bottle of wine, find a time when you aren't going to be disturbed and talk to your other half about where your sex life is right now. Take tissues; there may be tears. From either one of you – or both. If you just aren't enjoying it any more, you need to tell him. If you'd like a bit of time out to get your head around things, tell him. If you'd like him to be more patient with you, explain why, and how you feel. This isn't a blame thing; it should be an open conversation. You will get hot, and awkward, and embarrassed, but unless you want things to stay as they are, it's a conversation that you *need to have.*

The menopause makes you feel more sensitive about *everything*: criticism that comes your way, your body, how you think you look, how you think *they* think you look! A lot of what's going around in your head may not be happening in his, so keep that in mind. Explain that you aren't feeling like you used to and try to find a way for you to work through it *together.*

Step three. Is your libido low in your head or in your body? So, you've talked things through and shared the load, and everyone is on side, making sure you feel supported, loved and not put-upon. You still can't get revved up, though. It's probably time to have a blood test done to check your hormone levels, as they have may have taken a dip. Your GP will be able to arrange this and, once you know what you're dealing with, you'll be able to make an informed decision about what to do about it.

If your hormone levels are low, HRT is an option, and you can discuss what could work for you with your GP. If you'd prefer not to do this, there are natural alternatives which can lend a helping hand: meditation to improve your energy levels and calm your mind (see Chapter 6); vitamin and mineral supplements to boost your body, and foods to boost your mood (see Chapter 7); and exercise (see Chapter 8).

Step four. Work together and alone. It takes two to have sex, but it only takes one to have great sex. I'll explain . . .

You know how to drive a car, right? You drive the car every day and you probably don't give much thought to how it gets from A to B – it just does what you ask it to. Switch the ignition on, put it into gear, point it in the right direction and off you go. That's what sex can become like: a car that you drive to get you from A to B, without much thought or effort. It does what it's supposed to.

Now, imagine that over time, without you really noticing, parts of your car have begun to change, in the way that you only notice when you're driving it. Take the smear that your wipers leave on the windscreen, for example – you really must get them changed! But by the time you've got to where you need to be, switched off the engine and carried on with your day, a smudged windscreen isn't really on your mind any more.

Next thing you know, the radio station that you always listen to won't tune in properly . . . It's annoying but, after a while, you get used to the static and kind of zone out, hearing just enough of the songs to hum along to them, even if you can't quite hear what your favourite DJ is saying any more. The petrol light then comes on, and you know you should fill up but, well, it's cold and dark outside, and surely you can keep going for a little while longer? One day soon, you'll get in the car, and not only will you not be able to see where you're going, but the damn thing will have stopped working altogether.

If this happened, would you never drive again? If you'd be happy to stay at home, then great! Staying in and not having to change out of my slippers is one of my favourite things to do in the world. Although it does get a bit, well, lonely sometimes.

I know it's an effort to book the car in for a service, and to get the small jobs done – there are a hundred reasons to put off doing anything about the smudge, the staticky radio or the lack of petrol. (In fact, if we're carrying on with the petrol analogy, then we all know that feeling of pulling away from the pump, quietly relieved that we won't have to do that again for a while!) But with a few minor adjustments the smudge will be long gone and you'll be able to see clearly again. Sometimes all it takes is a little twiddle with the knobs and the radio communication becomes crystal clear. And with a full tank of petrol you can keep going and going and going . . . A word of warning, though: the longer you take to do something about things, the more difficult they will be to fix.

That's what losing your libido is like. You just feel . . . meh. What's the point? Some of the thoughts racing through your head might be that it's going to hurt, you're not going to enjoy it, you're going to take too long to come, and he'll just get bored and frustrated. You'll be embarrassed and, God, the whole thing will be such a bloody nightmare that you wish he'd just leave you alone.

But remember when it *wasn't* awful . . . ? Maybe, just maybe, it can be like that again . . .

A little 'me' time

One of our *Loose Women* guests has been Meg Matthews, who came on the show to talk about her experience of going through the menopause. She's started a website – megsmenopause.com – and it's well worth a look for a modern woman's take on what it's like to have the whole core of your existence turned upside down and inside out. It's further reassurance that you're not the only one feeling anxious and confused, comfort eating and hiding away from the world! Meg was extremely and refreshingly open about how she has dealt with her change, and one of the things she talked about with frank honesty was masturbation to help vaginal dryness.

I hadn't come across this and, judging by their reaction, neither had the audience or the press! It was fascinating: people were shocked that she had spoken so openly about something that most women do but few will admit to. Men joke and talk about masturbation freely enough, from sniggering teenage-boy chat at the back of the classroom through to pub banter about watching porn, but most women simply don't discuss that kind of thing amongst themselves.

I looked into the theory and, sure enough, on medical menopause sites and personal-experience forums for women going through the menopause, masturbation is listed as one way to help maintain the elasticity of the vaginal walls and keep the natural lubrication flowing. I didn't know this! Seeing as discomfort during intercourse is one of the main reasons why women go off sex, as a completely natural and cost-free exercise it's surely worth a try.

Apparently, masturbation is also good for boosting a flagging libido, as it reminds your brain and body what it's like to feel 'sexy'. Now that does make sense, as we all know that the longer we go without something, the less we feel like doing it – whether that's going to the gym, filling out your tax return or having sex.

So why not give it a go? You can even multitask. Lock the door, run a bath, slap on a face pack and off you go – who cares what the real reason is behind your healthy glow and the spring in your step, as long as it works!

HRT and your sex life

Women often ask me what kind of HRT I'm on. I've been prescribed four different therapies – oestrogen gel, which I rub on my skin daily; testosterone gel, which I apply once a week; oral progesterone tablets, which I take every night; and an oestrogen pessary, which I insert twice a week – and each serves a different purpose.

The oestrogen gel helps with many things, including low mood, and the testosterone gel is to improve energy levels, the development of lean muscle mass, strength and, importantly, sex drive. Many people don't think that women need testosterone but we do, especially if we've had a full hysterectomy and our ovaries have been removed. I take progesterone tablets, like other women who've had a hysterectomy for endometriosis, to prevent any endometrial tissue from becoming thickened under the influence of the oestrogen, and the oestrogen pessary alleviates vaginal dryness and thinning of the vaginal walls, both of which can make sex not merely uncomfortable but downright agony. How on earth can you relax and enjoy sex when you know it's going to hurt? I say this from first-hand experience and it's really important to do something about it, trust me.

If you're experiencing pain during intercourse, then this is where having a supportive, loving partner is not just a nice thing to have, it is *crucial*. It comes back to the confessions again: you need to talk to your other half about what is happening to you, and explain that things have changed down there.

Dry conditions

If you prefer not to use HRT, then lubricant is essential, otherwise . . . Oh my God, I'm wincing just thinking about it. You'll end up sore during and after sex, probably tearful and possibly resentful, which is not good for any relationship.

During the menopause your skin is likely to have become more sensitive as well, so normal lubricants might irritate you. Trying something that is water-based and hormone-free is a very good idea, and thankfully there are more brands than ever on the market, as manufacturers are waking up to the fact that there are legions of women in need. Sylk – which is marketed as a natural intimate moisturizer – is apparently good because it's both water-based and hormone-free, and can be bought in chemists or online, as can other brands such as Yes and Replens.

I think the main thing I've discovered along the way is that getting through the menopause is all about trial and error. As I think we're all aware by now, it's not a straightforward thing where there is one problem, one symptom and one solution. Symptoms and personal stories vary, and what works for one woman might not work for another. There is no 'quick fix' to make it all go away. It's about trying a little bit of this and a little bit of that, finding what works for you, and eventually it will all come good. The key is to do *something* to improve the situation.

It's just like sex. It's never going to work or get any better if both of you lie there not talking about what feels good or not so good, gritting your teeth and putting up with it! So talk, confess, and share ideas and experiences. It's the only way to find out what might just work for you. You only get one life, so you may as well do what you can to make it feel good.

Yes . . . yes . . . yes!

While we're on the subject of feeling good, one of the interesting things that very few people talk about when becoming perimenopausal is the rush of hormones that actually make you *want* to have sex. It's quite logical if you think about it; it's the body's way of saying, 'Get on with it! This is your last chance to get pregnant! Do it! Do it now! Do it again just in case!'

I'm pretty sure this was exactly how Victoria Wood was feeling when she sang 'The Ballad of Barry and Freda (Let's Do It)' with such gusto. I've never been able to look at a *Woman's Weekly* in quite the same way since hearing about Freda yearning to be beaten on the bottom with it . . . If you don't know the song, go and google it now. I'll wait – trust me, it's worth a quick timeout.

So while many women talk about their libido dropping through the floor as their body starts to change (which we now know is because their hormone levels have altered), there are others who are fizzing with the last flush of fertility!

It's so much easier to talk about *not* feeling like having sex and groaning about partners who do, because a) that's what everyone else is doing – or seems to be doing, and b) well, to own up to feeling frisky, with a skip in one's step, is flaunting it a bit. Isn't it a bit braggy? And no one wants to be friends with a smug so-and-so who's swinging from the chandeliers while you're feeling sluggish and low.

It's a bit like having a friend who's lost weight constantly telling you about the pair of jeans they just 'slipped into', while you know that, hidden under your jumper, the top button of your jeans is about to pop with the strain. It's not nice. So I think perhaps *that's* why we don't hear about this side of the perimenopause. We are British, and no one likes a show-off.

It is a thing, though. Your body's hormone levels fluctuate as you enter the menopausal stage, and some go up while others go down. It's also one of the benefits of HRT. So yes, having your hormones regulated to control the mood swings, night sweats, memory loss and other symptoms can also bring about the return of your libido – something you might have forgotten you ever had! What a pleasant surprise.

The 'manopause' (aka the andropause)

Bear in mind that most of us going through this stage in our life will be with partners who are of a similar age – anywhere from late forties onwards. If your partner is a woman, then it stands to reason that she will be experiencing similar physical and mental struggles. If your partner is a man, then brace yourself, so will he.

OK, it won't be exactly the same, but studies show that men also go through their own version of the 'manopause', called the andropause, where they get the same 'perimanopausal' rush that some women do – a need to seed, if you like. This can show itself in a good way, with a renewed vigour behind closed doors – which, of course, may or may not be welcome. However, if you're unlucky, it can also mean the purchase of an impractical car; hideous, inappropriate new clothes; or a lascivious look in his eye.

But what if you like it and they don't?

When you're going through a big drop in libido, it can be a lonely place to be. I was perimenopausal when the novel *Fifty Shades of Grey* first came out. I read it. I even made it to the end – and yes, my teeth were clenched at the atrocious Anastacia-isms and inner-goddess references, but I was curious to see what all the fuss was about. Everyone was talking about it – you couldn't sit on the tube without seeing ladies glued to their hardbacks or discreetly reading their Kindles. The media was going mad about sex: everyone was at it! We were all bonkers about bonking! And yet . . .

Something about it stayed with me. An uneasy feeling. Underneath all the huffing and puffing from friends, and the 'Huh! I *need* a blindfold to have sex with my other half – have you seen the state of him?' was a quiet, nagging issue which didn't quite ring true. It was one that I eventually raised with my friends on a night out – or rather a night in (I don't go out much) – and the response was not so much a whisper as a resounding pop of a cork being pulled. Followed by an outpouring.

I asked them what they thought about the antics of Mr Grey. At first, they said the same as everyone else: 'Huh!' As if they'd be up for all that messing about! Their own partners were lucky if they shaved their legs for them once a week, never mind any of that energetic stuff! However, a few glasses of honesty juice later and the truth flowed out.

It transpired that actually their partners *weren't* asking them about this crazy book that had taken the world by storm. The *men* were huffing and puffing about how stupid it was. *They* were hiding behind newspapers at breakfast, taking refuge in sports on the telly and letting rip with exaggerated yawns at the end of each day to send out the subtle-but-stinging signal that they weren't interested in sex. Not even a little bit. All this talk from women about 'fighting them off every week' or 'letting him have his way once a fortnight just to keep the peace' . . . For these women it was the other way round.

One tearful friend admitted that she hadn't had sex for

months because her husband was always too tired or stressed and just didn't seem to fancy her any more. He kept doing that 'I'll be up in a bit' thing at bedtime, and seemed to wait until he knew she was asleep before lying down softly, as far away from her as possible, and stiffening in all the wrong ways when she wrapped her loving arms around him. He was doing all the things that women do when their sex drive has dropped through the floor; he clearly loved her, but he just didn't 'want' her any more. The rejection was unbearable for her.

That same evening, a close friend admitted that she'd been told by her doctors that she was officially perimenopausal – she had the blood tests to prove it. She choked up as she told me the signs had been there, she just hadn't wanted to acknowledge them. However, now it was there in black and white, she had to do something about it, and that's what was scaring her. She'd spent the past year skirting around the issue of sex with her husband, being a loving and supportive wife in every other way, but freezing whenever he tried to initiate intimacy. He was very understanding of her excuses – they'd just moved house, she'd changed her job, their son was anxious about going to a new school. All these things made sense as to why she'd been feeling stressed and distant, but she knew the real reason was that she no longer had a sex drive, and didn't want him anywhere near her.

I felt so sorry for both my friends. Their sex lives were definitely grey, but not of the kind being gasped at by readers.

It makes me sad to think how many of us are going through this. I've been on both sides of the fence – and both are horrible! I think we *all* go through changes and, if we're ever going to get ourselves back on track, then we need to talk. I know how hard it is when you have to raise a tricky subject with someone you love, but if something is making you unhappy at your core, then why carry on pretending the problem's not there? Be honest. You may be surprised by the response you get. It could be the start of the best kind of change.

Sex after a hysterectomy. Will you ever do it again?

Another of the things women sidle up to me and ask about having had a hysterectomy, is 'What is the sex like afterwards?' I was at an event recently and, on the way to the loos, was ambushed by a very friendly lady who'd heard I was writing a book about the menopause. She told me how she'd cried and punched the air with joy back when I announced on the telly that I was having a hysterectomy. At last, someone in the public eye was talking about it! She was in her forties and, for medical reasons, had had to have a hysterectomy too. It had sent her into the menopause instantly, which she hadn't been prepared for, and it threw her off balance for a while – as it would anyone.

She went to her GP and was prescribed HRT (the gel kind), which she started rubbing on to her skin every day, and gradually found her way back to herself. Once her physical symptoms eased and her mind became more balanced, she realized that not only was she back to her normal self again, she was *better* than normal! Before her operation, she had spent three out of every four weeks of the month bleeding. Her periods were drawn-out and painful. How she'd managed to have four children, work and sustain a happy relationship was beyond me; I was exhausted just listening to her! Having a hysterectomy and going on HRT was life-changing for her. With no painful, draining periods to worry about, and her menopause symptoms dealt with, her energy and her libido began to rocket.

She laughed as she told me her husband now calls her the Martini Girl, as she's up for it 'any time, any place, anywhere . . .'

The first time . . . How soon is too soon?

For me, around four weeks after my operation I felt ready to try the one thing I'd been told to stay clear of: sex. Just the thought of letting Nick anywhere near my poor broken bits was enough to make me cross my legs. A month was a long time for us not to be intimate, though, and I missed the closeness of it, even if the act itself seemed a scary prospect. I liked the cuddling and the feeling of being close to him. Nick was a wonderful nurse and had spent those four weeks following the operation making sure that I was OK in every way, but I wanted to feel like 'me' again. I wanted to feel like 'us' again.

It was me who initiated it, one night as we got into bed. We were both as nervous as first-time teenagers. Would it hurt? Would I bleed? As he took his lead from me, it was impossible not to squeeze my eyes shut and grimace . . .

It was only when I tried to open my eyes again that I remembered I'd taken one of my strong sleeping tablets before getting into bed. My right eyelid stayed drooped and shut. I was getting sleepy and even though my mind was willing, my body wasn't on the same page at all. The medication was doing its job very well, and no amount of willpower was going to stop it! I tried to focus on the matter in hand, but my eyelid remained firmly closed and I could feel the other one starting to drop too. I wasn't thinking about what was happening down below at all – I was focusing every bit of energy on trying to open my eyes and not fall asleep on the job.

I quietly asked Nick to stop, and glanced up at him as best as I could. He looked so worried that I burst out laughing. I told him what was happening, reassured him that I wasn't having some kind of stroke, and we decided enough was enough. He gave me a hug, turned out the light and kissed me as I fell into a drug-induced stupor.

A week later, we tried again. We were both still nervous, but ready for it. We had some wine to try to relax, and tried to take our time and not think about 'it'. There were lots of things we could do to be intimate without actually having sex, we reasoned. So we started off slowly. Like a born-again virgin, my first time post-hysterectomy wasn't like something you see in the movies (especially not in *Fifty Shades . . .*). It involved fumbling, wincing, grimacing, waiting for pain, wondering if I would get wet enough so it wouldn't chafe, bracing myself for how it would feel when he was fully in, then trying to breathe out and relax enough to actually enjoy it. It took a while and lots of patience, and a concerted effort to focus on what felt nice rather than what *might* not, but we got there eventually. Both of us.

It worked. It was still a bit tender but, all in all, I'd say it went very well . . . So much so that within twenty-four hours I was sipping cystitis powders mixed with water, then had to get antibiotics from the GP, my face blushing furiously as I explained the situation. I hoped this wasn't going to be the norm from now on . . .

I do have to say that for a long while afterwards it actually did become the norm. I got urine infection after urine infection, and for days after having sex I would feel a dull ache like

I'd been kicked from the inside. I kept cystitis powders in the bathroom so I was always ready, and started taking cranberry tablets to calm things down.

Why, you might ask, did I carry on? Well, because sex to me is more than just the act of intercourse itself; it's about closeness and love. And it wasn't as if I didn't *want* to have sex – I did. I just had to deal with what was happening afterwards. Not having sex, or putting it off all the time because of possible pain, meant I didn't feel like Nick and I were as close as we could be, and I missed it.

Love hurts . . .

Things have never got back to how they were before, in the way that sex after having a baby is never *quite* as it used to be either. You simply can't think of your body in the same way; it doesn't feel exactly the same and, for most of us, certainly doesn't look the same.

While the urine infections and pain aren't as frequent now, they still feature. The pain doesn't just come after sex, it happens during it as well, which at times has made it difficult to relax and enjoy what's happening. It's like trying to have sex when you know the kids might not yet be quite asleep and you're listening out for creaking stairs . . . I know that at some point it's going to hurt, and although most of me is having a lovely time, a part of me has her teeth clenched waiting for the discomfort to come. It feels as if I'm being hit where my cervix used to be, like things are lower down than before. Afterwards my bladder feels sore, in that way it does before a urine infection starts.

As usual, I made a huge mistake and googled my symptoms,

and the most likely cause given was a prolapse. I looked into solutions and came across horrifying stories about poor women who'd had a transvaginal mesh inserted to treat the condition and who'd suffered terribly afterwards. Mesh is also a treatment for stress incontinence, which is so common after childbirth and during the menopause. I lay awake in bed for weeks worrying about all this; should I do something about the pain, or accept that it was better to live with it than risk an operation that could leave me debilitated and in agony?

I went back to see Mr Jan, who examined me and said everything looked OK. He said the most probable cause for my pain is adhesions from my hysterectomy, as I've suffered from them before. My bladder is most likely stuck to the scar where I've had my cervix removed, and this is what's causing the pain. The solution is a laparoscopy and adhesiolysis, which is a procedure that will separate the two, and a special gel will be put in between them, so they don't stick together again.

On the one hand I'm hugely relieved that I don't have a prolapse and don't have to consider the dreaded mesh. On the other, I'm reluctant to have yet another operation. I spoke to Nick about it and since then we've tried to work around it in our own way, by not going in as far, so nothing gets banged. It can be a bit distracting, and means I have half a mind waiting for it to hurt so I can say, 'Not so much!', which does kind of ruin the moment. However, now I know what the actual problem is I'm less worried about it, which is a huge help in itself.

Talking about the state of your sex life rather than putting up with any problems is the *number one* bit of advice I can give you. Sex is supposed to be something that makes both parties feel good and, if you're in a loving relationship, it has the potential to be one of the most emotionally connecting experiences you can share. If you can let someone put their penis inside you, you should also be able to talk to them about how it's making you feel. If it hurts, say something. If you can't find a way to work around it without it still hurting, go and see your doctor.

If you're too shy to see your doctor, get another doctor. There are a couple of GPs at my surgery with whom I'm much more comfortable talking about intimate things, so I'll book an appointment to see them rather than anyone else, even if it means waiting a few weeks. It's worth it. No one can help you if you don't tell them what you need help with! So stop procrastinating and start to deal with the issues that aren't working for you.

Dr Peers Says . . .

COMBATING VAGINAL DRYNESS

Due to the declining levels of oestrogen the menopause brings, the tissues in the vulva and vagina become thin and lose elasticity. There's less lubrication in the vagina and the consequent dryness can lead to painful sexual intercourse and risk of damage to the vaginal walls. The result may be loss of sexual desire as it's difficult to feel motivated to have sex when you know it's going to hurt. Almost two-thirds of women experience problems with vaginal dryness after the menopause but embarrassment and the inability to talk about it means that very few seek help.

The good news is that something can be done about it! Using vaginal oestrogen, either as a pessary or cream, restores the elasticity of the vaginal walls, increases the blood supply to the area, increases the production of secretions, and maintains acidity by lactobacillus colonization, thus making the vagina healthy and sex much more comfortable. Local oestrogen also stabilizes the bladder and reduces the need to get up and go to the toilet during the night, as well as helping with the sensation of an irritable bladder.[1]

WHAT'S BEHIND THAT FRISKY FEELING?

As we know, levels of hormones, including oestrogen, start to go up and down as we transition through the menopause. We mostly talk about the decline of oestrogen levels, as this is the cause of many of the unpleasant symptoms we encounter. But for some women, oestrogen levels can increase and lead to increased libido during the perimenopause due to ovulation occurring more frequently. As the perimenopause comes to an end, ovulation starts to decline and oestrogen levels then start to fall dramatically.[2]

THE ANDROPAUSE – FACT OR FICTION?

The term andropause is used to describe a 'male menopause'; however, this can be misleading. It suggests the symptoms such as depression, loss of sex drive, erectile dysfunction and other physical and emotional symptoms result from a sudden decline in hormones, in this case testosterone, but this isn't accurate. Although testosterone levels do decrease with age in men, the decline is steady – less than 2 per cent a year from around the age of thirty to forty. Unless there's a testosterone deficiency, due to a condition known as late-onset hypogonadism, the symptoms that men experience in midlife are unlikely to be due to hormones. Potential physical causes of such symptoms include lack of sleep or exercise, poor diet, smoking and alcohol consumption. Other factors that can contribute include work or relationship issues, money problems or concerns about ageing parents.

The condition Low Testosterone Syndrome (sometimes called Low-T) is easy to exclude and treat. I'd recommend an annual testosterone blood test (which must be taken before 10 in the morning) for men from the age of forty.[3]

TRANSVAGINAL MESH

Transvaginal mesh was an approach to the treatment of pelvic organ prolapse, where one or more of the organs in the pelvis slip down from their normal position and bulge into the vagina. Both synthetic and biological meshes were introduced to support the vaginal wall and the pelvic organs when previous treatment had failed or prolapse recurred.

Although treatment was successful for many women, there were reports of complications with their use. These included pain, incontinence, constipation, sexual problems and injury to the bladder or bowel. As a result, use of transvaginal meshes is now considered to be high risk and they're not recommended.[4]

ADHESIOLYSIS

Adhesiolysis is a procedure where adhesions, the bands of scar tissue that can form following surgery or result from infection or endometriosis, are cut and released. A biological barrier is then inserted between the bands to prevent reoccurrence. The procedure is carried out either via keyhole surgery (laparoscopy) or abdominal surgery (laparotomy). The former approach is generally preferred as it's associated with a lower rate of adhesion re-formation.[5]

1 Source: Women's Health Concern. Fact Sheet: Vaginal dryness. www.womens-health-concern.org

2 Source: Jean Hailes Foundation. About the menopause. www.jeanhailes.org.au

3 Source: NHS UK. Male menopause. www.nhs.uk/conditions/male-menopause

4 Source: NHS UK. Pelvic organ prolapse. www.nhs.uk/conditions/pelvic-organ-prolapse

5 Source: Reproductive Health Group. www.reproductivehealthgroup.co.uk/adhesiolysis

5

V is for Vasculitis

Now, first things first, *don't panic* when you read this. What happened to me is unheard of – *it will not happen to you*. In fact, the specialist I went to see said that in all his years of practice he had *never* heard of a case like mine. So I hesitated over whether to include my experience of vasculitis here, because technically it doesn't have anything to do with the menopause. However, I decided that, as part of my story, it goes some way to explaining the anxiety I've experienced, and which still rumbles on today. I'll talk more about anxiety in relation to the menopause in Chapter 6, but this particular episode of physical illness changed my attitude to life – a lot.

While it's hugely frightening to be diagnosed with a potentially life-threatening disease, living with the fallout pushed me to becoming more proactive and productive than I've ever been before. It hit home that you really do only get one life. I didn't want to look back on mine and wish I'd been brave enough to do something that was within my power to do, but a fear of failure held me back.

I have a framed quote by the poet Erin Hanson on my office wall, given to me by Nick and which sums up how I've tried to live my life since my diagnosis. It says, '"What if I fall?" "Oh, but my darling, what if you fly?"' and is just one of the reasons that you're holding this book in your hand right now – it gave me the courage of my convictions to make the menopause a subject women shouldn't be ashamed or embarrassed to talk about, when there's so much that can be done to help.

A couple of months after my operation, at my scheduled check-up with Mr Jan, we chatted about this and that, and he asked how I was getting on. After going through the things I'd been experiencing during my recovery and once he'd made sure I was healing well, I sat there smiling while he looked through the papers on his desk in front of him. He started his next sentence so naturally that the words took me by surprise.

'As you know, whenever we operate we test the tissue that is removed, and I have to let you know that the lab found something in your cervix.'

I looked at him uncertainly, not sure what he meant. I wasn't aware that anything *had* been tested.

'The tests found that you have something called medium vessel vasculitis. It's very rare.'

I laughed. 'I'm special, you mean!'

'Well, yes. Not many people even know about vasculitis. It's a disease of the blood vessels. What it can mean is that your blood vessels get blocked, and that can stop blood flow to your organs. Fortunately, my sister happens to be a vasculitis specialist, so I called her and we spoke about your case.'

He looked serious, and I stopped smiling. I began to feel cold.

'OK . . . What did she say?'

'Have you had any other symptoms of illness at all over the years? Other than your endometriosis?'

'Well, yes. I have a problem with my immune system, where I keep getting viruses. It's like shingles, but the doctors say it's not shingles. I get a rash on my torso, then my skin and muscles hurt so much I can't bear even the pressure of a cover on me. I get so exhausted that I have to take to my bed for days, sometimes a few weeks. It's happened for the past five years or so. I just thought I was getting really run down . . .'

'Well, that could explain a few things. It could be why you were in so much pain in your womb, because the blood flow to that area was being cut off. The good news is there's a chance that the affected tissue has all been removed now.'

'And if it hasn't?'

'I'd like you to have some blood tests to see if there are any antibodies in your system. That should tell us if we have got it all. Which would be great.'

'And that could mean that the other symptoms could clear up as well?'

'It may be the case.'

I wasn't sure how to feel. Was this good news or terrifying news? I stayed smiling and upbeat as I shook his hand and left to get my blood taken by the nurse. I went over and over the conversation in my mind as I headed home. Then I did the worst thing I possibly could. Again. I googled vasculitis. This was my diary entry for the next day:

There is no cure. I'm scared.

Had a dreadful night's sleep. I woke up many times soaked in sweat, roasting hot. Then woke up freezing cold when I'd tried to sleep without the covers on me. My mind went straight to my diagnosis. I don't want to be ill. I don't want to be a sick person. I don't want to be on steroids for the rest of my life, getting bloated and fat with bulging eyes. I want to look good, and keep my job, and have Nick fancy me when he looks at me. It's bad enough dealing with the menopause without this as well!

I got up this morning and, once the kids were at school, I spoke to Nick about how I was feeling. He completely understood and said all the right things, but it didn't help. So he sat me down, we got out our phones and headphones, and did a meditation together from the Headspace app.

As I sat on the floor with my eyes closed, I worked my way down my body, asking myself, 'How does my body feel?' My head felt tight, my jaw was clenched, my neck was cramped. My shoulders were rock hard, my stomach churning. My body was not happy. I then asked myself, 'How do I feel in myself?' and the words *anxious, frightened* and *distracted* came into my mind. When I asked myself, 'Why am I doing this today?' and the answer came, 'I am doing this to help me cope with my feelings right now', instantly I felt a little calmer. I focused on my breathing, counting one on my in-breath, and two on my out-breath. I did this until I got to ten, then started again. I did this over and over, focusing on how the breath felt as it filled my lungs, and how it felt when it left my body.

My mind was fluttering around, grabbing on to thoughts as they passed through: I needed to wrap Amy's birthday presents, I needed to get nibbles for the neighbours coming round tonight, I needed to sort out my website, I needed to do some writing, I didn't want to get sick, what if I got sick? As every thought came into my head, I told myself, 'Not now, I'm doing this . . .' and they drifted away.

As soon as one thought was replaced by another busy

one, I did the same thing, over and over again until finally my mind was still. As I breathed, I felt my neck give a quiet *pop* as it relaxed. I felt my jaw unclench. My shoulders fell away from my ears. My body stopped fighting itself. At the end of the ten minutes I opened my eyes. Ten quick minutes, and it had made all the difference.

I wrapped Amy's birthday presents, hid them in my wardrobe and got ready for the day.

When you have something like a hysterectomy, it stands to reason that you need to be braced for some bad news as well as good. After all, while they're rummaging around in there, there's a chance they might find something they weren't expecting. I must admit, this hadn't occurred to me; I was only thinking about what would happen to me after having my reproductive organs removed, not that they might discover I had some rare disease that had the potential to kill me.

Understandably, it made me re-evaluate things. It made me take stock of my life, my health, my relationship – everything. Well, it would, wouldn't it? I realized that while I was happy, there were lots of things that I either was just putting up with, or was putting off, and that needed to change. I suppose you could say it was a wake-up call.

I wrote down a list of the things that were making me unhappy, or that I wanted to sort out; the ambitions or dreams I had that I hadn't really pushed myself towards, either through fear or lack of confidence. Like so many women, I questioned my ability to do certain things, and tended to listen to that inner voice saying, 'Who the hell do you think you are, imagining you can write that book/do that job/be that successful . . . ?'

I needed to face up to the reality that I held myself back subconsciously because I was scared about what would happen if I actually *did* write the book/get the job/was that successful. What if after all my efforts, I discovered I actually *couldn't* do it? That I was a sham? That I'd fooled everyone for so long into thinking that I was capable of doing the work I did, but that was *all* I was really capable of doing?

I know that many people feel like this; that their livelihood might be snatched away at a moment's notice because people might discover they aren't really as good at their job or as talented as they appear to be. I felt it – I'd always felt it – and it has a name: imposter syndrome. The fear of being exposed as a fraud.

However, with the threat of serious illness hanging over me, I now knew that I couldn't let that mental hiccup hold me back any longer. I had to accept that it was all in my head. Women – particularly of a certain age – can suffer enormously from imposter syndrome. Have you felt this before? If you have, you can't let it hold you back either.

It doesn't mean that the fear will ever go, but we can learn to manage it and live with it. The menopause is called 'the change' for many reasons, some of which can be good, if you use it as a time to take stock and decide what you do and don't want in your life. It can be a chance to think about what you've already achieved in life, and what more is to come. What you have to believe is that there *is* plenty more to come.

So . . . I made changes. I left my agent and found a new one, who I felt could better help me achieve the dreams I'd kept inside. It's a scary move to make, because your agent is essentially your manager and handles all the jobs that come in for you, but they also work with you, to try to help you reach your full potential. It's an important relationship to get right, especially for a woman approaching fifty, who makes her living in the public eye.

In my agent, I needed someone to also see my capabilities. At my age you can either begin to stagnate, or you can push the envelope and start to challenge yourself. I chose the latter. I'd like to encourage you to do the same.

This might seem a trivial thing, but I decided to change my car, too. I'd been driving a Mini but decided to go for the kind of car I'd always wanted, even though it wasn't the most practical. (Sounds like a clichéd midlife crisis, doesn't it?) Now I had Nick in my life and was no longer a single mum, we'd become a two-car family, so mine no longer had to be a sensible one. So, I traded the Mini for a soft-top. Shiny and black, with heated seats, and a camera and sensors to help me park. It was all I'd ever wanted! It was definitely a 'seize the day' purchase, and I can't tell you how much joy getting into it every day still gives me. It's not the fanciest car in the world, but it's mine, and I love how driving it makes me feel. It's impractical, it's beautiful, and I love it.

I also stopped being afraid of saying what I wanted. This was a *big deal*. And I think it's a particularly big deal for women who often suppress their own needs in favour of those of the family. I have moments where I have flashes of confidence and think, 'Right, I can do this. I'm going to get out there and be amazing! I'm going to pitch ideas, stand by my convictions and achieve fantastic things – write novels, come up with brilliant programme ideas, put myself out there to try new things . . .' And then all of them get turned down, one by one, my confidence shrinks back to zero and I quietly go back to where I was, wondering why I ever tried in the first place.

When I got my vasculitis diagnosis I decided that I was going to keep trying, come what may. I'd been given a second chance, and I wasn't going to waste it. There's definitely a lesson for everyone there. Don't doubt yourself. Don't give up. Age is no barrier.

Re-evaluating your life is quite a common thing for anyone to do on receiving a diagnosis like mine, or any other illness for that matter. We hear the word *cancer* so often that we tend to think that might be the thing that will kill us, but there are so many ways to be unwell. And when you think life is coming to an end, you've never wanted to live so much.

When I finally got the all-clear, after months of tests on my organs, I was exhausted with relief. I still have to have regular blood tests to make sure it hasn't returned, but for now – touch wood – my vasculitis has been completely surgically removed and I am fine. The wake-up call has stayed with me, though. Life can never be quite the same again.

One of the biggest changes that happened in my life following my hysterectomy and vasculitis worries was that I got married! I think it's really important to remember that when we're going through an incredibly difficult time and trying to hold it together for our families – whether it's something like vasculitis or the menopause – our partners are also dealing with their own pain. All the worries that we have about ourselves, they also share. So when I got the all-clear, it wasn't just a happy day for me, it was also a huge moment for Nick.

I, of course, didn't realize this at the time, but he'd decided that as we approached the anniversary of our fourth year together, he wasn't going to wait to make our relationship permanent and binding . . . he planned to ask me to marry him. The proposal itself took me completely by surprise. Not because I didn't think he'd ever ask me – we'd discussed it, so I knew we'd get round to doing it at some point – but I guess I'd had other things on my mind.

It happened in Paris, on a short trip away, and I must admit that when we were planning our little holiday, a tiny voice in my brain thought . . . maybe? When the moment actually happened, it caught me completely unawares, however, because for the two days beforehand I had been a *menopausal nightmare*. I was all over the place. Edgy, snappy, irritable, angry, selfish, sulky . . . In essence, an absolute moody cow.

It had all come to a head. I'd said some horrible stuff, then cried, and we'd talked it all out and decided to draw a line under things and start afresh the next day. I was so surprised when he proposed, my face was a picture – literally. He took a selfie at the exact moment he popped the question, and I look a state.

Once I'd actually said yes, and we'd stopped crying, I asked him why on earth he'd asked me *then*? When I'd been such a nightmare? His reply was just one of the reasons why I know I've finally met the man who will be my partner for life. He said that he knew I wasn't myself, that I was clearly going through some kind of moment. That once we'd talked things through and he knew I still loved him and we were OK, he still loved the person that I really am, even if he wasn't too keen on the person I had been during my 'moment'.

You can't put a price on a partner who understands that how you behave when you're being ruled by your hormones is not representative of who you really are. It isn't easy to live with a menopausal woman – even when that person is you! For all the HRT, vitamins, exercise and fresh air in the world, the strongest medication is love. True support keeps you going when those other things don't touch the sides. I'm not saying love and support can replace the appropriate medication and alternative treatments – hell, no! But without love, wherever it comes from – friends, family, a partner – life can seem ever so much darker. I'm so thankful that I have someone in my life who brings me light. I hope you've got someone by your side, too.

Dr Peers Says . . .

VASCULITIS

Vasculitis means inflammation of the blood vessels. It develops when the immune system attacks healthy blood vessels and causes them to become narrow and swollen. It's a rare inflammatory disease affecting approximately two to three thousand people in the UK each year and can be a minor complaint, affecting just the skin, or a more serious illness that causes heart and kidney problems. There are three main causes of vasculitis: an acute reaction to an infection, drug or chemical; a secondary reaction to another illness such as rheumatoid arthritis or cancer; or occurrence as a primary disease, unrelated to any other illness. Treatment involves the use of drugs that suppress the body's immune system and control the inflammation.[1]

1 Sources: Vasculitis UK. Understanding vasculitis. www.vasculitis.org.uk; NHS UK. Vasculitis. www.nhs.uk/conditions/vasculitis

6

It's Not All in Your Head

'Anxiety attacks – awful. I felt like I was dying.'

'Confusion, not wanting to go out, loss of confidence,
feeling as if my mind and body have been taken over
by an alien being.'

'I feel like I'm going mad! My confidence has
plummeted and I cannot sleep. I'm a strong person
but I feel needy and wish it would be over soon!'

'If you want to conquer fear, don't sit at home and
think about it. Go out and get busy.' Dale Carnegie

The menopausal paradox

I read a brilliant book recently called *The Chimp Paradox* by
Professor Steve Peters. It's all about how we have two brains –
our rational human brain and our chimp brain – and that's
why we behave the way we do in certain situations. It's a great
book for helping you understand not only your own reactions
to things, but also the reactions of others. So the next time
someone barges in front of you at the supermarket, or you're

cut up by an aggressive driver, it really helps to think, 'Ah, that's their chimp', and not take it so personally.

It got me thinking that as well as having parts of our brain that react in certain ways to different situations – causing feelings of happiness, sadness, stress, anger, and so on – as a woman, and particularly a woman going through intense hormonal change, there is also a 'female paradox' at play.

Ever since I was a young girl, I've always been the type of person who wants to do well. I like to do things properly, colour within the lines, get my homework in on time. I've always tried to do the right thing. So, how do you feel, and what do you do, when you're doing everything right but it still feels like it's all going wrong? Because that's what the menopause feels like.

Things that used to work just don't any more. Sleep has become the final frontier. Pain, in various forms, has become the norm. And anxiety – off-the-scale fear and dread, paralysing terror, a rumbling inside that rises up so that you feel sick and your skin, teeth, hair and eyes hurt – has taken up residence. At its worst, during a panic attack, I feel as if I'm swelling – ballooning – and that my mouth is becoming a gaping hole in my head. How do you function when you feel like this? How can this be 'normal' and just accepted as part of 'the change'?

I know I'm predisposed to anxiety because of my personality type – these feelings are nothing new to me but they used to surface infrequently. I used to have a panic attack – quietly and wordlessly – in the passenger seat of the car every time my ex-husband drove us to see his mother, for example. It was like drowning on land, in full view, but nobody knew it was happening except me. Now they happen all the time – still quietly and neatly without me making a fuss – but happening none the less.

My GP has been amazing. She understands and supports me. In the past, I've seen male doctors who, I'm sure through gentle ignorance rather than insensitivity, haven't been as understanding of the female condition. How is it possible for a woman to be strident and strong in her professional life, capable and loving as a mother, compassionate and passionate as a partner, and yet sob with inconsolable sadness and desolation at how wretched and inadequate she feels? This, to me, is the female paradox.

We've all felt a bit low at times, or worried about things, but depression and anxiety are more than feeling a little sad that things aren't going your way. In fact, some of my most stressful and anxious times have been when *everything* has been going my way. When life is grand and things are sorted – what the hell is there to be worried about? That's actually when I worry about everything.

What is menopausal anxiety?

It's well documented that low mood and feelings of anxiety, helplessness and anger are key symptoms of the menopause – and I've contended with them all, as have you, I'm sure. They're just some of the rainbow colours of emotions that make us human, and I fully understand the need to experience shade so that you can appreciate light. However, I also know that these feelings have grown in me over the past few years, and I believe that's down to hormonal change.

In my experience, depression during the menopause is similar to postnatal depression in that you're aware that you're not feeling yourself, but you can't remember what 'yourself' feels like any more. I think lots of women feel this way, and just try to carry on. However, just as a woman who has had a baby is not the same as she was before, neither is a woman going through 'the change'. Hormone fluctuations have affected you, as has contending with all the psychological issues surrounding the menopause, such as body image, sexuality and ageing.

Taking HRT or vitamin supplements will help you have more good days than bad, but if you really feel as if you're spinning out of control, talk to someone. Your GP may be able to recommend someone (a therapist, if you both think that will help), or something, to you. It might be as simple as trying a herbal remedy such as St John's wort – multiple studies have found that this is helpful for depression – and making some lifestyle changes (see Chapters 7 and 8), or you might need an antidepressant for a while.

However, first and foremost, talk to your friends about how you're feeling; you'll be surprised how many of them are feeling the same way. And if they judge you, *pffft*, what kind of friends are they?

I'd also recommend keeping a diary of everything that you're feeling mentally as well as physically, so that you can see for yourself if there's any kind of pattern to your moods. It could flag causes you hadn't considered. Could it be something about your job, a person or a situation that's making you feel stressed, anxious or depressed? Sometimes when something (or someone) has become such an entrenched part of our existence, we don't see that it (or they) is actually causing us to feel ill. This realization can be life-changing.

It can be as small as someone who constantly puts you

down, makes little digs that eat away at you, undermines your confidence and hurts your feelings. It's like death by paper cuts; each one is so small and seemingly inconsequential that to mention it might seem petty. But over time, these little cuts add up and while there's little to see on the outside, the internal wounds are deep and raw. A diary can help you see where these little cuts are coming from, and with the help and support of people who love you, you'll feel more able to speak up about how these things are making you feel. That in itself will go a long way towards making you feel better.

I've always suffered with low moods, but have managed to overcome them (in part, on a day-to-day level – not when they've been at their worst) through a combination of exercise, diet, fresh air, setting goals and trying to look on the bright side. A positive mental attitude really can take you a long way. However, with severe depression, looking on the bright side doesn't cut it. No amount of 'pulling my socks up' or thinking, 'What have I got to be depressed about?' is going to help.

Despite problems with low moods, I'd still describe myself as a naturally optimistic person. If a problem comes up, I'll always look for a solution. I don't dwell. I enjoy being nice to people. I like asking them about their day, about themselves, and making them smile and feel good. I get a lot of pleasure out of that. I've realized over the years that actually, sometimes it's when I'm at my most unhappy that I try to make other people happy; to distract myself from myself. I'm both sides of the coin.

Nonetheless, I've always been an anxious type. Not that anyone would know. I've largely kept it to myself and just cracked on with things, pushing myself forward, smiling, keeping busy . . . Underneath, though, there's always been this rumbling unease. It's a bit like when you're standing in a building and can feel and hear a tube train passing beneath your feet. It's not a big deal – it's just a train, right? But it feels strange, knowing it's there, rumbling underground in the dark, making us tremble, even as we stand in the light.

In the past, anxiety wasn't something that I ever spoke about, because I didn't know how to put what I was feeling into words, so I pushed it down instead. Every now and then it would rear its head and roar, like a monster I didn't want to acknowledge I lived with. Then it would eventually pull its head back and retreat into slumber. I'd hope it had gone for good, but deep down I'd know it was still there, and that one day it would be poked awake again.

I've always worried about stuff. Anything. Everything. Real stuff that is worthy of a sleepless night, but also things that can very easily go away and sort themselves out. When I was growing up, I moved around a lot with my family, and while my little sister seemed to handle each relocation with breezy ease, I was angst-ridden and crippled with self-doubt. At a new school, there's one sure-fire way to make sure no one wants to be friends with you, and that's to walk in midway through the year and be announced as the new girl, which is what happened to me over and over again.

I tried too hard to hide how frightened I was and, as a result, managed either to scare everyone else away with my weird cheeriness, or was a magnet for bullies. It was enough to make anyone anxious. In my adult life, in terms of my inner workings, not much has changed, but I'm better at hiding my fear. Most of us become better at pretending everything is absolutely fine.

Since going through the menopause, however, this anxiety has taken on a life of its own. And I know I'm not alone in this. Anxiety now paralyses me. It swallows me up. I can't think straight, or focus. I'm convinced that I'm stupid, ugly and unloveable. I can't sleep at night or function during the day. It weighs so heavily on me sometimes that I can't breathe.

So, anxiety is something I know a lot about. I think I'll always experience it to some degree, and I have to confess that just reading this book won't make any of your symptoms go away. That would be a bit like buying a diet cookbook and expecting to lose weight just by having it sitting on your shelf (come on, *we've all done it*). Rather, this is an opportunity to share what I've experienced, and what works for me, in the hope that it might work for you, too. It doesn't mean the various strategies I employ do the trick 100 per cent of the time, because I don't practise what I preach 100 per cent of the time. I fall off wagons, I forget, I'm lazy. Like you, I'm a human being. I do work at it, though; I try to keep it under control.

I know that meditation works and even though I don't always feel like it, I do it. I switch on my app, stuff in my earphones, and breeaathe . . . It doesn't eradicate those anxious feelings completely, and sometimes I can barely hear the instructions over the thud of my pounding heart and the grinding of my teeth, but it does help.

I also do yoga, on my own, in my bedroom. I very rarely go to classes as I never seem to be able to fit them in around work and childcare, so I do the stretches on my own – again listening to an app – and eventually I'll feel myself calming down. On other occasions, I go for a walk and get some fresh air, if I feel able to leave the house. Yes, really. Some days even stepping outside my front door is too much to ask, and I'll only do it if I really have to – for work or the kids. If it was down to me, I'd stay inside, light my lovely-smelling candles and pretend that I've stayed in out of choice rather than necessity.

So there are several things you could try to help manage your anxiety – you don't simply have to live with it.

Get scribbling

I find that writing things down helps my anxiety a lot. This might be because I'm instinctively a polite person and can't bring myself to say out loud if I'm feeling cross, or if someone is *seriously* getting on my nerves. In order not to scare everyone off, I prefer to put things down on paper. I often write in the Notes section of my phone, but you might want to invest in a journal instead – there are plenty to choose from. Gratitude or happiness journals work for some people, helping to focus the mind on the good stuff, but sometimes all you need to do is vent.

Although I've been assured that my severe resting bitch face lets the world know when I'm *not* happy, I'd beg to differ – people don't know the half of it! I wrote the piece that follows to let off some steam one day as my kids played in one of those indoor water parks. It's one with slides they can whoosh down and fountains they can splash in. I'm not a great fan of standing around in my bathing suit, baring my cellulite to the world and pretending I'm loving the deafening screams and splashes to the face. I enjoyed it when they were little tots, and I got as much joy as they did; seeing their chubby little arms and legs thrash around in the water, grinning their gummy smiles from ear to ear. But now that they're older (mine are teenagers and in-between-agers), I'm far happier letting them get on with it while I sit down with a coffee, waving from afar. One day in the not too distant past I sat with my coffee and my laptop, and I wrote this . . .

Nobody likes a stinky bin

I've got one of those fancy bins. It's stainless steel, tall and sleek, with a black click-top. I can open it with my elbow when my hands are full of stuff, and the lid makes a reassuring cluh-clink before rising with slow confidence, like a butler opening a door and enquiring, 'You rang?'

I use it countless times a day, and I take it for granted as it stands in my kitchen. I don't give it a second thought – it's just there, doing what it's supposed to, until the lid doesn't quite shut unless I push down all the rubbish inside. With the final load – the one that refuses to be squashed and compacted – the stink finally hits me: the foetid smell of discarded daily detritus; stuff that is now starting to reek.

I also own another metal box: a lovely shiny car that zips along nicely. I was in it today and, not for the first time, I shouted at another driver. A man zoomed towards me on the wrong side of the road, even though I had right of way, and didn't acknowledge me when I had to brake sharply to let him through. I was furious, honked my horn angrily, and yelled a few choice words at him.

The man's car screeched to a halt, and I could see him staring at me in his rear-view mirror. He was clearly angry. I was cross too, but he looked as if he might actually do something about it, rather than do what I do, which is to squash my anger down.

You see, every day my rage is pushed down and kept

in check, manifesting itself in Walter Mitty-like daydreams of witty retorts, shouting rude words, or occasionally punching someone really hard on the nose. Because I would never actually do anything; it all goes on in my head. The raging, the clenched-jaw mutterings, the stomach-churning, ulcer-inducing thoughts of violence – they don't ever come to anything.

I do wonder what life would be like if I could actually say what was bothering me at the time, rather than stuffing it away with all the other irritants in my internal Room 101. If I was able to say out loud, clearly and without flinching, what I really thought. Passive aggression is my forte, you see, because I don't have the nerve to be assertive. That would take actual courage, and carry the risk of someone shouting back at me or, even worse, giving me the thump on the nose that I would dearly love to give them.

I'm so consumed with pent-up fury that sometimes it leaks out of me like a stinky smell. You see, when I honked my horn at that driver, I realized that my bin and I have a lot in common.

On the outside I might look as if I've got it together, but click open my lid and I'm a decaying buffet of petty grudges and bite-sized irritations, mixed together with putrid dollops of fear and self-doubt. Some of these are legitimate issues that deserve their place in this pit of emotion – past experiences that were horrible enough to warrant their odorous funk. I've dealt with them the best way I can: squashing them down to the bottom so that no one else can see or smell them.

I know that the best thing to do would be to take myself to the tip, and dump the lot of it, but that would involve looking at what's inside. I'd be forced to examine everything I've crammed away and dredge up memories. I finally understood today that what stops me doing that is the fear of being overpowered by it all, because, actually, I'm afraid that it's stronger than me.

So, the question is: is that OK? Probably not, but here's the rub. Life is good right now. It's sweet. So do I tackle something I can't see – and only occasionally feel – just to know that my metaphorical bin is clean? I deal with my life as it is now, I try to be present in each moment, and enjoy the good while I'm experiencing it rather than focusing on the bad. For me, that involves pushing unpleasantness down and dealing with it at some point in the future.

I'd rather have a little clear-out every now and then, and put a nice clean liner on top of the blackened, bonded-to-the-sides rot. Those are the bits that need scrubbing until I'm sweaty and wished I hadn't started. No one notices them anyway. Don't we all have them? Some issues will need soaking for years in the gentle, soapy water of therapy before they can be wiped clean away. Others are just part of the fabric of life – problems, frustrations and annoyances that come with just existing in the world.

It doesn't matter who we are, we have rubbish thrown at us every day, and that is as much a by-product of life as the stuff we chuck away ourselves. Some people keep that rubbish in a bucket under the sink, others put it straight into a wheelie bin outside. My bin stands tall for all to see: it might be sleek and competent, but open it up and it stinks like any other.

I wrote this just before my hysterectomy when I was full to the brim of horrible memories from my past and anxieties about my future. I was pushing things down, but I accept now that you have to allow these feelings to the surface in order to deal with them properly. Never more so than when you're menopausal.

Writing the piece gave me the release I clearly needed at the time – I felt better just getting it out of me. In this instance, it came out as a piece of prose about a metaphorical bin, but for you it can take any form you like. Bullet points, poems, long ramblings, jumbled-up thoughts that make no sense to anyone but you – it doesn't matter. If you can't let it out, get it down.

Give yourself some headspace

I've spoken about the medical route I've taken to make myself feel better over the years, from antidepressants to HRT, both taken for good reason and both immensely helpful. But mindfulness is something I came across a few years ago that has genuinely changed my life. I know it's very 'of the moment' and everybody seems to be talking about it and jumping on the mindfulness bandwagon, but there's a reason it's so popular. It works.

It sounds pretty bonkers, making yourself sit still and giving your mind a rest for ten minutes or so, but I can't stress enough what a good idea it is. My mind is full to the brim of nonsense most of the time, and I'd hazard that yours is too. From petty arguments that leave me rummaging around my brain for a pithy comeback long after the event, to worries about life, love and everything else in between. I can keep my brain very busy, having looped conversations with myself that mainly serve to stress me out even more. So anything that helps me quiet my mind is a *good thing*.

I have my meditation app, but there are also some brilliant books on the subject, from small-format ones that you pick up at the till in gift shops, through to the fantastic *A Mindfulness Guide for the Frazzled* by Ruby Wax. I'd really recommend Ruby's book if you'd like to know more about how the mind works, and how much benefit mindfulness and meditation bring to an overactive brain.

Mindfulness is all about paying attention to the present moment and it's recommended by the NHS as one of their five steps to improving mental well-being. Yes, you'll certainly feel calmer but recent research has also shown that it has a biological impact on the body. Scientists have found that an eight-week mindfulness course can help lower levels of inflammatory markers and stress hormones in the body by around 15 per cent. It's free and feels like a really acceptable way of de-stressing, and helping you to manage your stress better, to be more resilient.

I started off doing mindfulness sessions just sitting on my bathroom floor, as it was the only place I could get any peace and quiet for long enough. These days I'll sometimes do it once the kids have gone to school and I'm alone in the house, but other times I have to do it on the hop – literally on the train journey to work in the morning. It's not the same experience but it still does the job.

There are lots of apps and techniques out there that are useful for first-time meditators. Insight Timer is a good one if you like to have tinkly music in the background. The app I use, called Headspace, works best for me. I find it useful to be guided through what I'm doing. It keeps me on track and stops my mind wandering so far off that I can't get it back again – and I like the sound of Andy Puddicombe's soothing voice. He's the co-founder of Headspace, and has written books on mindfulness, too.

Meditation for beginners

You can, of course, practise mindfulness without any help. If you want to try it on your own, this is what you do:

• Find somewhere quiet to sit, where you won't be disturbed for at least 15 minutes. I think mindfulness is most effective when done in the morning, as it sets you up well for the rest of the day, but do it whenever and wherever works best for you. And don't think, 'Oh, it's too late, I've missed my chance today, I'll do it tomorrow.' It's never too late.

• You can sit in a chair or on the floor – wherever you're comfortable. I like to lean against something otherwise my back hurts. You don't get extra points for being a hardy sort, so I'd recommend that you do the same. Don't sit on a squishy sofa or tuck yourself up in bed, as there are also no prizes for guessing what happens then, and nodding off is not the same as meditating.

• Set a timer for 10 minutes. I'd recommend the one on your phone as it will count down silently. A kitchen timer ticking away next to you won't do at all. If you can set the alarm to a gentle sound, such as a soft chime, then do that. You don't want to be jolted out of your state of relaxation by a piercing buzzer.

- Get yourself settled and comfortable – you'll be sitting still for a while. Rest your hands on your lap. You don't need to place them in any special way, just however suits you.

- Start by taking a few deep breaths. Getting some air deep into your lungs clears your head and you'll be amazed at how much better you'll start to feel. Despite the fact that we do it from the moment we're born until the moment we die, most of us are rubbish at breathing. Make sure to inhale deeply through your nose, and out through your mouth.

- When you've done this a few times, close your eyes, and let your breathing return to normal.

- Pay attention to the sounds that you hear around you and familiarize yourself with them so they don't disturb you. It sounds crazy, but something as simple as acknowledging, 'That's a dripping tap. That's my neighbour's dog barking. That's a delivery van reversing . . .' will stop them from becoming petty annoyances that prod you in the face while you're trying to relax. You've acknowledged them, they have nothing to do with what you're doing right now, so let them go.

- Start to scan your body, from the top of your head down to your toes. Focus on what each part of it feels like, but in passing; don't dwell over any niggles. I have a permanently stiff neck after three unfortunate and quite serious whiplash injuries, so my body scan goes something like this: 'My head is fine, my face is fine, my neck is stiff, my shoulders are sore, my arms are fine, my hands are fine, my chest is fine, my stomach is sore, my thighs are fine, my legs are fine, my feet are fine.'

You can use whichever words work for you, this is only an

example. Just make sure to comment on how your body feels in a matter-of-fact way, not lingering over any discomfort. You're not having to do anything about any aches, you're just recognizing them for what they are and moving on. Even just saying the parts of the body – and you don't have to do it out loud – works for me as well: 'Head, face, neck, throat, shoulders, arms, elbows, forearms, wrists, hands, fingers, back, chest, stomach, lower back, pelvis, buttocks, thighs, knees, shins, calves, ankles, feet, soles of feet, toes . . .' Work your way down in whichever way feels right for you.

• Ask yourself, 'Why am I doing this?' and not in a grumpy way. I tend to say to myself, 'I'm doing this today to make me relax, to help me cope with things better.' Other times, I'm doing it because I'm feeling stressed, or low, or anxious. Or because I want to be a more patient mother and partner. Sometimes I say I'm doing it because it feels good. There are no rules.

• Then ask yourself, 'How do I feel?' Now this is interesting. Usually, we're so conditioned to reply 'Fine', we don't really ask ourselves how we're feeling at any one moment. We might be trying to hide the emotion (annoyed) or enjoy it (happy). However, we don't really own up to it or put a name to it. No one is going to hear you, though – this is just for you – and I can't tell you how liberating it is to say, 'I'm pissed off today. I'm in a really bad mood', when you've just done the mum thing and smiled and waved your kids off to school, or had a really bad day at work. Be honest. Say to yourself, 'I'm feeling grumpy today. I'm stressed today.' No one is going to judge you.

It can be just as liberating to say, 'I'm feeling calm today. I'm feeling happy.' You're not trying to change your emotional state or do anything about it, and you're not trying to impress anyone. Having done this, you should be feeling a little more relaxed.

• Start to focus on your breath again. Feel the air coming in through your nose, going down into your lungs. Notice how your chest feels when it expands and contracts, as the air passes in and out of your body. Do this a few times, and then start to number each breath, counting 'one' as it goes in, 'two' as it goes out, and so on. Do this until you get to ten, and then start over again.

• Now that sounds very simple, but it's actually where the mindfulness bit starts to come in. While you're counting, it's very likely that your brain will decide it would rather drip-feed an annoying tune into your head, and you can't *quite* remember who it's by. Then you'll remember that you forgot to buy that birthday card you were supposed to. Or get Weetabix. And who was it you were going to call this afternoon about that funny smell coming out of the plughole in the bath? And, oh God, that's right – the dentist. You were meant to book that six-month check-up for the kids. Now their teeth are going to rot and fall out, and it's all your fault. What number was I on again . . . ?

You get the gist. This is where the breathing and the counting come in, though – to give your mind a rest from all this stuff. It's all important, obviously (especially the irritating song by . . . who is it by again?). You just don't need to think about it right now.

So when your mind starts to wander – and it will, every time (this bit doesn't stop happening, you just get better at stepping away from the chatter) – I like to think of these unwelcome thoughts as being a bit like pesky kids. Think about this from a grown-up's point of view. You know when you're in the middle of doing something and a child rushes up and tugs your arm because they *must* show you a) a stick they found; b) the hole in their sock; or c) their favourite YouTube clip of a cat? You're right in the middle of a) a phone call to work; b) cooking dinner; or c) a juicy bit of gossip from a friend. In any case, you're busy, so you can't stop and admire the stick, hole or cat. So you say, 'Not right now – in a minute.'

If you're the kind of parent who drops everything the moment your child sneezes, then this method may not work for you, but I'm quite good at saying, 'Not now – in a minute' to mine, especially if the reason is c) some really juicy gossip. You haven't said, 'No, go away! I will not listen to you, stop it, I won't look . . . *aarrgghh*! I'm looking! I've forgotten where I was!'

However, that's exactly what happens when you try to force your brain to ignore the annoying thoughts as they pop up, tugging on your mind's sleeve and demanding instant attention. Instead, you say very nicely, 'I know you're there, but I'm doing *this* right now. I'll see to you in a minute.' The pesky thought, rather than hanging on to your arm and whining until you pay it some attention, will then wander off to draw on walls or flush things down the loo, or whatever it is thoughts do while no one is paying them attention.

I find that the pesky kids analogy works because that's what thoughts are like. They flounce around in your brain like hyperactive toddlers wanting someone to play with, and just need a bit of parental guidance.

• So, when you're breathing in and out, and counting, and a thought pops in, acknowledge it, but don't stop what you're doing. Recognize it for what it is: it's a thought and you'll deal with it later. If it helps, you can even say in your head, 'That's just a thought'. It will drift away, then, sure enough, another thought will arrive. Keep breathing and counting, acknowledge this new thought, then let it pass too.

•   Random feelings will also rise up – who knew so much could go on in your head while you're just sitting there, minding your own business, breathing in and out! They're rarely happy ones, but if they are, then excellent – they can stay. However, sometimes a thought can pop into your head which will remind you of something that made you angry. So now you feel anger. I like to think of such emotions as moody teenagers. As with the thoughts, though, simply acknowledge them for what they are, all the while breathing and counting.

It sounds like an awful lot of work, doesn't it? But here's the thing. If you weren't meditating, you'd still have all those thoughts and feelings mooching around your head anyway, but you'd have them while you're trying to get on with your day and cope with the things that really need to be dealt with. It explains why, at the end of each day, you feel knackered and ratty with everyone – your brain is worn out from sorting out real stuff on the outside, and nonsense on the inside.

Practising mindfulness is your chance to let your brain have a rest and switch off for a while. When it does, amazing things happen to your body. Your stress levels drop, as do your stress hormones. Even if you only manage to get to ten a handful of times, your mind and your body will feel the benefit. If you do it every day – just for 10 minutes – it will get easier, because you'll learn how to shush the annoying thoughts and feelings. It won't work every time; some days the thoughts will keep banging on and on, and you'll have to stop counting and give in to them. That's fine. Try again later on, or the next day – don't beat yourself up about it. Sometimes the kids win. But eventually they'll learn to play on their own for a little while.

• When your timer goes off, let your mind wander for a few moments. Don't think about counting or about your breath. Your mind will probably be quite happy just to stay where it is and will sit quietly in your head, awaiting further instruction. After a few breaths, tune into the sounds around you. You'll be amazed at what you blocked out while you were busy focusing on your breath – the dripping tap and neighbour's dog were there all along.

Bring your focus to your body and start to notice how heavy it feels: the weight of it pressing into the chair or the floor, your hands in your lap, your head on your shoulders. Again, you'll be astonished how you hadn't noticed them before. Slowly open your eyes, and allow yourself to readjust to being back in the room. Think about how you feel now. However that may be is OK. There's no right or wrong. Once you feel ready, slowly get up and carry on with your day.

That's it. It's simple but it can be tricky, and you do need to persevere with it. Trust me, though – it works. It won't make all your troubles go away, or make you 'better', but it really will help.

Even though I do it every day, I still get moments where I'm so swamped by anxious thoughts that I think I'm swelling to twice my size. My face starts to prickle and I can't feel my hands. The logical part of me knows that those physical symptoms are a reaction to how I'm feeling. I'm getting pins and needles because I'm not breathing deeply enough. My brain tries to rationalize it, but it doesn't always work. Sometimes all you can do is stop and allow it to happen. However, while your brain is going haywire, try to remember that you do have the tools to make yourself feel better. The menopause is a bumpy road, and the changes your body is going through will not always sit comfortably with your mind. Knowing there are little things you can do to take the edge off how awful it can make you feel is one way of making your journey through the menopause smoother. It doesn't mean that the issues will all go away. But *it will pass*.

When the wheels come off the bus

The wheels came off my bus when I was feeling particularly stressed about my upcoming wedding. The big day had grown and grown in my head until it was all I could think about. It made me ill: my nerve endings felt as if they were severed, my skin hurt to touch, my jaw ached from being clenched, and it was like I was losing my mind. I kept going to work, I functioned, but the *second* I was on my own – even if I just nipped to the loo – the feeling I was going to implode swamped me.

One morning – after another terrible night's sleep where I'd woken at 2.30 a.m., only to lie there worrying and stressing about everything going on in my life, and even things that weren't – I was on my way to work on the train. It had just gone 7 a.m. and I was packed in with all the other commuters. I was lucky enough to have bagged a seat, which was fortunate because I felt awful. I was exhausted. I felt rough. And then I started to feel a panic attack building.

It started off as prickles – the horribly familiar sensation I get on my face and scalp that tells me an attack is on its way. I tried to breathe deeply and calm myself down, but it was like trying to stop a speeding car by standing in front of it and waving. My feelings mowed me down. Nausea surged up from my stomach and hot, bitter bile filled my throat.

By now I was gasping for air and had to take my coat off, despite the early morning chill in the carriage. I gathered my bags and stood up, lurching past the other passengers to get to the door. The train pulled in to a station and as the door opened, I fell out and onto the platform, before moving away from the throng. I found a seat and sat down heavily, my elbows on my knees and my head down, as I breathed deeply. 'Please don't throw up, please don't throw up' was all I could think.

I sat and breathed, and breathed, and breathed. Eventually, I recovered enough to raise my head. Then I felt tearful and stupid as well as sick. I couldn't go to work. I was so frightened that I'd either throw up or fall down. What if it happened again while I was on live TV and the whole country saw what a mess I was? I couldn't do it. I got my phone out and texted Emma, our deputy editor, and told her I'd had to get off the train as I wasn't well, that I was really sorry but I was going back home. I felt guilty and weak and annoyed with myself.

I made my way out of the station slowly and hailed a cab back home. The kids were still asleep but Nick was up and looked surprised when I let myself into the house. I explained what had happened. He took my bag and coat off me as I cried uselessly, then led me upstairs to bed and tucked me in. The next thing I knew, it was midday. I had slept and slept. My body and mind had crashed. I spent the rest of the day in bed while the world carried on without me.

And that's the key thing to take from this: the world carried on without me.

It's OK to stop

We all like to think that we're vital to the running of our families' lives – let's face it, we usually do most of the rushing around, picking up and sorting out, don't we? I was so consumed with planning the wedding and making sure that the kids were happy with how the day was going to be that it all got on top of me. My other worry was that Nick's and my relationship would fall apart once we got married, and that my heart would get broken again. Nick pointed out gently that while my previous marriages hadn't worked out as I'd hoped, I hadn't been married to *him*. So this time would be different. And he was right.

The world will keep turning if we stop for a while and take a mindful moment or two. Sometimes our bodies and minds have to go further than just tapping us on the shoulder and whispering, 'I'm really not feeling myself . . .' before we take any notice. Listen to your body, and to your mind. Sometimes you'll end up crashing before you can bounce back up again, and other times you might catch yourself mid-fall.

Know yourself. And let those who love you know what's happening, too. You don't have to do this on your own. The world isn't going to stop challenging you just because you're menopausal and a bit fragile. So you have to be kinder to yourself.

Dr Peers Says . . .

TACKLING DEPRESSION AND ANXIETY

Accurate statistics regarding the number of women affected by depression or anxiety during the menopause are difficult to track down. However, research suggests that 1 in 10 women may experience depression at this time. Some women may be more prone to developing it than others, especially if they've experienced episodes earlier in their lives. For all women, the effects of hot flushes and night sweats on sleep; negative beliefs about the menopause and ageing; and the busy lifestyles and demands of midlife can increase the risk of depression.

Oestrogen and progesterone naturally inhibit anxiety and work together with receptors in the brain to help you cope with stress. As the levels of these hormones begin to decline, anxiety can become a problem and lead to panic attacks if left untreated. Certainly, many women I see suffer from, and describe, severe anxiety and feeling anxious, sometimes for no apparent reason at all. This can be extremely alarming as it seems to come from nowhere!

For some women, HRT can help with symptoms of anxiety or depression occurring during the menopause. When they persist, cognitive behavioural therapy (CBT) or a course of antidepressants may also be helpful.

CBT is a talking therapy focused on helping you manage your problems by changing the way you think and behave. It's based on the concept that your thoughts, feelings, physical sensations and actions are all linked. By breaking down these thoughts and feelings into smaller parts, the negative patterns are disrupted and problems become less overwhelming. Unlike other talking therapies, CBT looks for practical ways to improve your state of mind about current problems on a daily basis rather than dwell on issues or events from the past. The National Institute for Health and Care Excellence (NICE) recommends CBT as a way of alleviating many menopausal symptoms including anxiety and stress, depressed mood, hot flushes and night sweats, sleep problems and fatigue.

If your symptoms are more severe, or fail to benefit from approaches such as CBT, you may be prescribed antidepressants. These work by increasing levels of the chemicals in the brain, known as neurotransmitters, linked to mood and emotion. Treatment usually lasts for at least six months, or may be longer if you have a prior history of depression or experience severe symptoms.[1]

THE MEDICINE OF MINDFULNESS

Mindfulness is about being present in the here and now. It involves paying attention to your breathing and how your body is feeling; being more aware of approaching thoughts and feelings and reacting differently to them. Menopausal symptoms such as night sweats, hot flushes and irritability can all feel worse when you're feeling stressed. Focusing on your breathing for 10 minutes can have a positive effect on how you feel, allowing you to become calmer and control your thoughts regarding the negative effects of the symptoms. I personally use an app to help me meditate called Calm, which describes and teaches mindfulness.[2]

1 *Sources: British Menopause Society. Cognitive Behaviour Therapy (CBT) for Menopausal Symptoms. www.thebms.org.uk/publications/factsheets/ cognitive-behaviour-therapy-cbt-menopausal-symptoms/; Menopause Health Matters. Menopause and panic attacks. www.menopausehealth-matters.com; NHS UK. Clinical depression treatment. www.nhs.uk; NHS UK. Cognitive behavioural therapy (CBT). www.nhs.uk; Women's Health Concern. Mood symptoms. www.womens-health-concern.org; Depression Toolkit. Menopause. www.depressiontoolkit.org*

2 *Source: Mindfulness UK. www.mindfulnessuk.com/mindfulness-the-menopause*

7

How to Eat

'I'm eating tons of soya beans in the hope that I can naturally increase oestrogen levels. Apparently, Japanese women do not suffer the menopause like we do – they eat a lot of soya. Worth a try!'

'I've cut out caffeine as that makes my anxiety worse. Cut down on sugar. Try to have a green juice a day. Take vitamins plus cod liver oil to help joint pain.'

'I know that coffee and chocolate make my hot flushes worse but I just can't give them up.'

As I fell headlong into the menopause and approached my hysterectomy, I decided to re-evaluate my diet. It was 100 per cent *not* to do with losing weight and everything to do with getting my body ready for life-changing surgery. I wasn't looking for a faddy regime – for me, it was, and remains, a lifestyle change.

I'm not going to get preachy and tell you off for eating cake or enjoying a cheeky glass of *vino* (who doesn't love cake and wine? What's the point of *living* without cake and wine? How much harder would the menopause be without cake and wine!). No, I took certain steps to make sure I could look back after I'd had my operation and know, hand on heart, that I'd done everything I could to help my body to get through the surgery and heal afterwards.

When your body is going through huge changes, taking the time to look at the food you're putting into it makes a lot of sense. It can be difficult to feel healthy when you're menopausal, but your diet has a big impact on how well you feel. If you've never given it much thought before, now's the time.

When it comes to the food we eat, we all go through different stages during our adult lives. The first is when you leave home and have to fend for yourself. In my case, that meant surviving on chips, cider, and pasta with tuna. Then, in my twenties, it meant living on stir-fries and heartache, with white wine thrown into the mix. I became a mum in my thirties and with having to cook for a family came the realization that I couldn't *actually* cook and no one liked my food.

That was when I started cooking only what the family would eat, because there's nothing on earth more demoralizing than spending hours preparing home-made, organic, made-from-the-heart fare, only to have your kids spit it out. I know that back in the day they'd have been forced to sit there until the wee hours of the morning, until they'd eaten every last bite, but I just let mine go to bed with rumbly tummies and grumbly mouths.

Cooking became all about limiting expectations (mainly my own), and my priority was to prepare food that was fresh, healthy but primarily palatable for the short people in the house. I stopped thinking about what I liked or what might be good for me; mealtimes came down to whatever was easiest to make and caused the least fuss.

As the menopause approached, I reached yet another stage; one where I had to start thinking about my needs. The time had come to feed my body and mind the foods they need to thrive.

How to feel good naked

When I started looking into food as a source of health, rather than just fuel, it felt a bit self-indulgent. I know that's an utterly ridiculous and back-to-front way to think, but realizing that I was eating to feel good not look good was huge for me. In a way, mindful eating is how to *feel* good naked, rather than how to look good . . . but the upside is that you *will* look good naked. Even with surgical scars, stretch marks and all the wobbly bits that we women have.

Having said that, our weight, whether we like to admit it or not, can be a huge factor in how we feel about ourselves. Whether or not you've struggled with your weight in the past, either with putting it on or not being able to gain it, dealing with it now is different to at any other time in your life. During the menopause it can creep on, slowly and quietly round your middle, and refuse to budge. When even supermodels like the beautiful Yasmin Le Bon admit to getting a 'layer of padding all over' (*Red* magazine, March 2018), you know that any weight gain we might battle during our hormonal change is completely normal.

Feeding our body what it needs at this time in life, and getting it right possibly for the first time ever – certainly in my case – is a world away from chips and cider. Also remember that if you're looking into changing your diet because of a hysterectomy, you've had major surgery, your body is knitting itself back together, and your hormones are all over the place. It's different to recovering from *any other* operation you will ever have. Anyone who has had a knee op and says they know what it feels like needs a firm poke in the eye. They don't have a clue.

You need a lot of self-care and a well-balanced diet. Bear in mind that 'well balanced' means different things to different people, so while we're all recommended to eat plenty of fruit, vegetables and protein (and plenty of fibre if you're having a problem with constipation), our bodies react individually. We literally stomach things in our own way, so find what works for you. I personally can't eat too much fruit as it gives me a tummy ache, and I'm not keen on red meat. So I eat lots of veg and fish because they agree with me. I'm intolerant to dairy, so I use almond milk and soya spreads rather than cow's milk or butter. But that's just me and my stomach. If you're thinking of radically overhauling the way you eat, always consult your doctor first, to make sure you're going about it the right way.

Am I what I eat?

I'm not a dietician but there are some good suggestions here for how you might consider eating differently and better in order to have a more manageable menopause. I'm going to share with you the changes I made before my operation, and what making them did for me, physically and mentally.

First of all, a couple of months before my operation, I looked up what foods are good for different needs. It made sense to me that some foods would be beneficial during the menopause, because magazines are always full of articles telling us that we should be eating oily fish for one thing and leafy green veg for another. I just needed to find out what might help someone about to have her hormonal tap switched off at source.

As much as anything, I was interested to find out what foods might stop me from going mad. I was just as worried about the mental side effects of having a hysterectomy as I was the physical. I still am. Having experienced depression before and knowing how horrible it is, if I can do anything at all to stop it coming back to the point where I'm really struggling, then I will.

I think we have to be honest with ourselves about this. Most people will feel depressed from time to time; it's part of our human nature not to feel on top of the world at all times. That kind of euphoria is unsustainable. Even rollercoasters need to dip so they can rise. Clinical depression, however, is very different to feeling mildly depressed. Just as anxiety is different to feeling a bit stressed. These feelings eat away at you like acid on skin; you just can't see it on the outside. They are hideous and, having experienced both of them, I know that they both hover over me like invisible Dementors from *Harry Potter*, waiting to suck the joy out of me. So I take whatever natural steps I can to stave them off.

So, what to eat? Needless to say, a healthy, balanced diet is a good thing full stop. For a start, it'll help you to minimize any excess weight gain which might creep up on you during the menopause. It isn't inevitable but it tends to happen largely because you're not as active as you once were, because you may feel like comfort eating through all the grim symptoms, or because your metabolism slows, your hormones change and your body holds on to more fat. Carrying less weight can ease some of the symptoms of the menopause. Here are the basics:

• The main foods to cut down on are those containing saturated fats, sugar and salt. There are some foods that are good for menopausal symptoms, both mental and physical, and some that aren't – such as cake and refined carbs, caffeine and alcohol. Ouch. You aren't going to like this, but if you're suffering from hot flushes, then cutting down on your evening tipples and nibbles will make a huge difference. That means less coffee, and less of the wine, chocolate and spicy food in front of the telly before bedtime. Gulp.

• Iron is vital! It's especially important if you suffer from heavy bleeding when you have a period, as whatever levels you have will get depleted. Lentils, beans, dark green leafy veggies, baked potatoes, cashews, tofu, wholegrain bread and grass-fed red meat are all good natural sources of iron. It can be tricky for the body to absorb, though, so taking it in a liquid form works well – you can pick up bottles of iron-rich, energy-boosting brown gloop from most chemists.

• During the menopause, it's especially important to look after your bones to minimize your risk of developing osteoporosis, so make sure you're getting lots of calcium. Dairy products such as milk, cheese and yoghurt are all calcium rich. I'd stay away from any lower-fat versions as they tend to be crammed with sugar to make them more palatable. It's far better to eat smaller amounts of the real thing than kid yourself by eating loads of low-fat foods, whose added sugars turn to fat inside you anyway.

Green leafy vegetables are also good sources of calcium (with the exception of spinach, which also contains oxylates – natural compounds which bind with calcium, making it difficult for your body to absorb it), and that's probably why kale is having its moment. Try to snack on almonds, Brazil nuts and sesame seeds, and get a few portions of fish where you also eat the small bones, such as sardines, into your diet each week.

• Protein is brilliant for helping the body to recover from illness, so look for oily fish and lean cuts of meat, which you should grill or steam rather than fry. You can also get protein from eggs, pulses, beans, nuts and tofu.

When it comes to eating for the mind, I looked into what kind of foods I should be having to keep my moods as balanced as possible. Cutting out caffeine is important as it can send your hormones on a rollercoaster, but it's also a stimulant that affects the nervous system, triggering mood instability – so there's one more reason to cut your lattes down to one a day.

Complex carbs such as potatoes, bran and wheat are good for boosting your serotonin levels, which is necessary to help you function properly, as low levels can lead to depression, poor sleep and a reduced sex drive. Protein, in meat, soy or dairy form, is important as the amino acids in protein-rich foods have also been shown to help women cope with mood swings.

Food, vitamins and sex

I promised you earlier that I'd give you a list of vitamins and minerals that help with a flagging libido. The great news is that making sure you get enough of them in your diet will not only help to give you a boost in the bedroom but will also make you feel better in every way.

• **Vitamin D:** Have you ever wondered why you're a little more receptive to the idea of sex when you're on holiday? It's not just the heat, the swaying palm trees and cocktails that play a part (although they do!), it's also all the lovely vitamin D that you're getting from that big yellow ball in the sky. Here in the UK we have to hit the supplements to get those kind of levels during the winter months.

I personally find that oral vitamin D sprays work much better than tablets. The liquid form is more readily absorbed, and just a few squirts a day on the tongue can make a difference. You can find sprays online, or in most health food stores. Once you know what you're looking for, it's amazing what you find!

During the spring and summer, try to get as much natural sunlight as you can without putting yourself at risk of melanoma. Also, look out for oily fish again (it's always oily fish, isn't it?), egg yolks and red meat as sources of this much-needed vitamin.

• **Vitamin B2:** This plays an important role in lubricating the body from the inside, so if you need a bit of help with vaginal dryness, then try upping your intake of B2-rich foods, such as red meat, dairy products and mushrooms.

• **Vitamin B3:** This helpful little vitamin is what gives you the energy you need not only to have sex in the first place, but also the bursts you need to orgasm. Start adding tomatoes, peanuts and brown rice to your diet for a little extra va-va-voom!

- **Vitamin B12:** This is the vitamin that most of us are deficient in, and you'll know it if you're constantly tired, lethargic and not interested in sex in the slightest. Try eating more eggs, tuna, crab and clams. If you're vegan, you may struggle to get enough of this vitamin from your diet alone, so you might need to take a supplement or get a vitamin B12 shot.

- **Iron:** This is such an important part of our make-up, and is the one thing that most of us forget to keep on top of. Low levels can mean you don't feel like having sex, and you don't enjoy it much when you do. Iron is found in green leafy veg, such as kale and spinach, as well as grass-fed beef.

In addition to a bit of online research, I also asked around and got ideas from friends about how to start putting meals together. I'm not a cook, and I like food that's easy to prepare and doesn't need loads of unpronounceable and difficult-to-source ingredients. I normally don't think about cooking myself something to eat until I'm ravenous, and by then I'm well past the point of wanting to marinate something for hours, or even having to peel a mushroom. I want food – *now*! That's why for years I've existed on stir-fries, and was horrified to learn that the ready-made sauces I've been pouring happily over my healthy prawns and veg are packed full of sugar. As are my 'healthy' snack bars and my muesli. I'd been getting it wrong all this time and didn't even know! So I had to start again.

I'd also been using a NutriBullet (there are, of course, other blenders out there, this is just the one that I use). You stuff healthy fruit and veg into it, mix in some ground seeds and powders, then blend it all into a drink. The only problem was that over time I'd stopped making ones with vegetables because they all tasted like dirty dishwater. The last time I'd used spinach, beetroot and carrot, I'd vomited the whole lot up quicker than I'd swallowed it down. If that isn't enough to put you off a healthy lifestyle, I don't know what is.

So I'd been using it to whizz up the same drink every day: a milkshake made with banana, almond milk, cacao powder, flaxseeds, chia seeds, and a dash of agave syrup. A lovely drink. But not really the most virtuous to be having every morning, as it contains its fair share of calories.

I'm sure that using blenders to fix healthy drinks every day is very good for you. I can't seem to stomach the super-healthy ones, but if you can, then it makes sense to give it a go. I just have to get my nutrients from eating vegetables rather than drinking them . . .

I won't lie, looking again at what I was eating was daunting, and I didn't even recognize a lot of the stuff I was expected to stock up on. Once I started, though, I realized that these ingredients had been there on the supermarket shelf all along; I just hadn't been aware of them. Lentils, miso paste, chickpeas, dates and nuts soon became part of my daily diet – along with my usual ingredients of salmon and green veg – and I found that once I got used to using them, they became as easy to prepare as my usual stuff. I just needed to make this new way of cooking as much of a habit as my old one.

Also, big confession here – I'm lazy, and I like to stick with what I know, because, to be honest, I can't be bothered to shake things up. However, with my impending operation and being in the throes of perimenopause, I needed to be bothered. In fact, I was at the point where I was really quite hot and bothered, and the whole diet shake-up was so that I didn't lose my mind and started to feel better in myself.

They're pretty decent reasons to push yourself out of your comfort zone.

Eating for the menopause

The internet is awash with recipes and books filled with recipes that can help ease menopause symptoms, which is useful but can also seem a bit overwhelming. For me, once I can cook something without having to look in a book to remind me what I need to buy from the supermarket and how to put it all together, *then* it will slip into my everyday life.

Now that you've read what foods are helpful, you could begin by simply adapting recipes you're already familiar with to include some of the key wellness ingredients. I'd recommend introducing more chickpeas, soy and miso (which are all high in protein), brown rice (which is so much better for you than white rice), salmon, mackerel and sweet potato (which is high in fibre and full of vitamins A and C). This can be as simple as putting a few handfuls of spinach and/or chickpeas in your favourite curry, swapping your normal baked potato for a sweet one, or your burger for a salmon fishcake.

As for things that are unhelpful to have in your diet, too much sugar and caffeine can send your hormones into overdrive, causing their levels to spike and drop. None of us experiencing the menopause needs that – our hormones are doing enough of it of their own volition; they don't need any extra help. So I started cutting back my intake of both. I reduced my coffee to one cup a day, and stopped quaffing a full cafetière of the stuff, with two heaped spoons of sugar in each mug (brown, obviously, because everyone thinks it's better for you). In my solitary cup of coffee, I replaced the sugar with a teeny squeeze of agave syrup because it *felt* like it was healthier. I also stopped buying biscuits that I actually liked, so that I wouldn't eat them. Our family had to make do without Jaffa Cakes and chocolate wafers, because if I couldn't have them then they couldn't be in the house!

I was doing quite well with my diet in the run-up to the op. The problems started when I was recovering afterwards and stuck in the house for weeks on end. I didn't have the energy to do all the things I normally do if I'm not at work: exercise, chores, running around after everyone else, getting stuff done.

When the biggest achievement I racked up during a day was moving from the sofa to the armchair and wearing a different pair of leggings from the day before, it was only a matter of time before the snacking started. *I like snacking.* It just doesn't like me. Or maybe it loves me, which is why the results wrap around my bottom and thighs, refusing to budge. I am, of course, not alone in this.

One of the things I'd noticed the most about cutting back on sugar (you'll notice I didn't say I cut *out* sugar; I'd be lying if I said I'd managed that) was that I wasn't getting as hungry. My energy levels were much more constant, not spiking and plummeting, leaving me ravenous and desperate for *anything* to eat, *immediately*. I got hungry for breakfast, lunch and dinner, and had a few little nibbles in between on walnuts and Medjool dates, but I wasn't constantly raiding the snack cupboard, staring at the Jaffa Cakes and drooling.

In fact, my craving for chocolate and biscuits fell away. Two weeks after my operation I was bought a box of chocolates for my birthday and I gave it to the kids. They devoured it in front of me and, hand on heart, I didn't want even one. That was *unheard of*.

What drove me to snacking was boredom. There's only so much sitting on the sofa, little walks and online shopping a woman can do before her tummy starts to rumble. (By the way, my lifeline throughout this whole experience? The internet. I'd have been ruined without my laptop, and not just because I did a lot of journalling about my experience while I was off work, which was good for my head. No, I ordered a whole new wardrobe, because I was going through a life-changing time, which *obviously* called for new clothes. I ordered new clothes for Nick and the kids, too. I bought a new bin for the kitchen. Literally, a new wardrobe for the bedroom. New sofas. I'm freelance, so when I don't work I don't get paid; I'm not entitled to perks such as holiday or sick pay. So being off work cost me a fortune, and that's without taking into account the fact that I wasn't getting paid. It's what I was spending online every day that nearly ruined me. But back to the snacking . . .)

My friend Nadia Sawalha had warned me that my addiction to Medjool-date-and-almond-butter balls was going to have me piling on the pounds – Nick and I were getting through handfuls of the neat little treats every night! (You can find the recipe on page 173, but brace yourself, they're more-ish.) I stopped making them, and instead sat in front of the telly with a packet of dates and a big jar of almond butter, smearing a date with some before shoving it into my mouth. Oh God. It was like snogging someone you really fancy but knowing he's not right for you. It felt so good, but I had to pull away before I stuck my whole head in the jar and ate until I was sick.

So, as I discovered, even snacking on good stuff can be bad for you (doesn't that sum up just how unfair life is?), but only if you eat too much of it. The health benefits of almonds are well known. They're rich in vitamin E, so good for the immune system and for fighting off bacteria and viruses, and also contain calcium, iron, zinc and selenium. They're so rich in nutrients they can help with diabetes, constipation, coughs, anaemia, and with hair and skin health. If you eat them raw – in salads and casseroles, for example – your body absorbs their nutrients even more readily. Amazing, right?

Dates are, of course, a great source of fibre. They also contain vitamins such as riboflavin (B2, which is good for migraines) and vitamin A (which is good for healthy vision and the immune system, amongst other things). However, they're also packed with sugar – so, moderation in all things (which is exactly why I didn't give up wine. Seriously. If I was going to have my womb and ovaries ripped out, my bladder and intestines fiddled with, my emotions battered and my brain frazzled, I figured that a glass of brutally chilled Sauvignon Blanc was the very least I deserved).

On the pages that follow, I'm including some of the recipes I used to get me on track, to give my body the nutrients it needed to help me through a tough time mentally and physically. They're simply the ones that I found useful, so please look around for others that suit you and your palate if these don't take your fancy. What I will say is that we all *know* that cutting the crap out of our diets makes us feel better. You don't need to be a rocket scientist (or a dietician) to work that out. So eating the foods that are recommended to help with hormone imbalances – almonds, seeds, avocados, broccoli, berries, pomegranates, beans, lentils, quinoa, bran, salmon and eggs – is bound to be a good idea.

Putting your new diet in place is the tough part. But stick

with it. The benefits are amazing. I've started with this recipe, as it's the one I loved the most then had to cut right back on. It comes with a warning – they are moreish!

Date and almond butter balls

3 tsp goji berries
15 Medjool dates, stones removed
4 dsp almond butter
4 tbsp coconut oil
3 tbsp raw cacao powder
1 tsp macha powder
2 tbsp almond milk
300g desiccated coconut

Blitz the goji berries and dates in a food processor. This can be a bit tricky; you might have to stop and start a bit until they're chopped up enough. Add the remaining ingredients, except the almond milk and desiccated coconut. Blitz again and add the milk bit by bit until everything comes together and forms a paste. You may need more or less liquid, depending on how dry or sticky the mixture is. You need it to be firm enough to hold together, but not too wet.

Divide the mixture evenly and shape into little balls (slightly smaller than a ping-pong ball is ideal, but really they can be any size you like), then roll in the desiccated coconut until covered evenly. Place the balls on a baking tray lined with greaseproof paper and leave in the fridge until hard – this will take a couple of hours.

If you keep them in a Tupperware container in the

freezer, they'll last for longer – weeks, even. Well, I think they'll last weeks. I've never personally been able to leave them alone that long. They'll obviously be frozen when you take them out to eat, so you can leave them for 10 minutes or so to soften a bit, or just get stuck in, whichever you prefer.

If you like, you could toast the coconut in a dry frying pan over a low heat, tossing regularly until the flakes start to brown. Don't let them burn, though – they'll taste awful and it's very annoying having to throw them all away!

....

My food diary

My typical food diary isn't perfect, and probably isn't balanced enough, but it's realistic. I'm not suggesting you follow it, but it might give you some ideas for how to adapt your own diet to make sure you're getting more of the nutrients and vitamins your body needs as it's going through the menopause.

.... *Breakfast* ....

For years the received wisdom was that breakfast is the most important meal of the day. After all, it's the meal that 'breaks the fast', so it stands to reason that you need to fill yourself up with hearty goodness to give you all the energy and nutrients to get through your busy morning. Now, however, the thinking is much more fluid.

Some corners feel that we should fast overnight for at least 12–16 hours, apparently to let our cells rejuvenate. While this can lead to weight loss, it can also result in reduced energy levels, heartburn, caffeine dependency, brain fog and headaches. All of which are already being experienced by menopausal women as we go through 'the change'. So, for me personally, I think having something to eat in the morning, even if it's something small, is a good idea.

In recent times, there's also been much discussion in the press about the importance of maintaining good gut health – not just to look after our digestive system, but for our overall health. I looked into this in more detail after my hysterectomy as I'd heard and read a little about it, but wasn't really sure what it was all about.

In a nutshell, around 60–80 per cent of our immune system is in our gut, and an imbalance there has been linked to imbalances in hormones, chronic fatigue, anxiety and depression, as well as skin problems such as eczema and rosacea. So it makes sense to me to include some kind of probiotic in your diet to boost your gut health. There are loads on the market – whether it's a tiny pot of gloopy drink or in tablet form – containing bacteria such as bifidobacteria and lactobacillus.

I try to get my probiotic intake from eating sauerkraut. Before you balk at the idea, hear me out. I've never been a pickled cabbage fan. To be honest, I'm not sure anyone is born a pickled cabbage fan, but once you get used to eating it every day, I'd go so far as to say it's actually quite nice. You can either have a few heaped forkfuls straight from the jar, or add it to salads. I have it with scrambled egg and smoked salmon on toast – sounds weird, but it works.

So why sauerkraut? Because it's full to bursting with probiotics and lactobacillus bacteria, which are great for your gut. It's also high in fibre, and contains iron and vitamins C and K.

Because of how it's fermented (with salt), it can also contain a fair amount of sodium, so don't get carried away and eat too much of the stuff.

Now, before you go rushing off to buy some, be aware that not all sauerkraut is created equal. The vinegary offering that's chucked on to hot dogs at half-time is not the same deal, as it's pasteurized to make it last longer – a process which kills off all the good stuff that you're after. Look for raw, organic sauerkraut that has been fermented using just salt, and hasn't been cooked or pasteurized. You can find jars of it in the supermarkets and health food shops – you just might not have noticed them before.

You can even make it yourself, if you like. It involves slicing up a white cabbage, putting it in a big bowl and rubbing in a tablespoon of salt with your hands. You then bash the cabbage with a pestle and mortar until water comes out, before squishing it all into a Mason jar and leaving it to ferment for between three days and two weeks. Or you could do what I do and just buy it and keep it in the fridge . . .

First thing in the morning, I also take a load of supplements – Menopace, zinc, vitamins C and D, and collagen – as well as applying my HRT gel. Generally, you're advised to take a supplement that includes vitamins A, C, D, E and the full spectrum of B complex vitamins (B1, B2, B3, B6, B7, B9, B12). But you really need to consult your GP about this, as they'll know what's right for you. It could be useful to ask for a blood test before you start taking any, to see exactly what you might be lacking.

Moringa tea. This is how a usual day starts. It was recommended to me as it's jam-packed with things that are good for your immune system. Made from the leaves of the tree *Moringa oleifera*, it's an invigorating drink full of nutrients and loaded with antioxidants. It's said to fight inflammation and can improve digestion, balance blood sugars, protect and nourish the skin, and help stabilize our mood. The list goes on. If I don't have any of that around, then I'll settle for a herbal tea: peppermint, green, ginger or camomile.

I'll have a few more cups throughout the day, along with so many glasses of water I lose count. If I'm out and about, I always have a bottle of water with me so that I don't get dehydrated – I use a reusable stainless steel one. I drink loads of the stuff and always have done. (And I still get spots – go figure.)

Virgin Mary. The perfect solution if I haven't got time for a 'proper' breakfast: tomato juice, grated or ground turmeric (which is the superfood of the moment; it's known for its anti-inflammatory and antioxidant properties), salt, pepper, lemon juice, Tabasco and Worcestershire sauce. Yum. All of these ingredients, where possible, are organic. It just makes sense to cut out of your diet as many unnecessary pesticides and hormones as possible, especially when yours are raging.

Banana smoothie. It's probably best not to have this every day, as it's quite calorific, but it's also jam-packed with good stuff, and perfect if you have a busy, active few hours ahead of you. Take your blender and add one banana, two heaped tablespoons of porridge oats, a teaspoon each of flaxseeds, matcha powder and chia seeds, a sprinkling of goji berries (I thought these were a load of nonsense when I first heard about them, but now I add them to soups as well as smoothies, and lap up the vitamins A, C and B2 they provide, as well as iron), a handful of blueberries, a tablespoon of peanut butter and a teaspoon of honey. Add a little almond milk and blend until smooth. Top up with enough almond milk to reach the right consistency and blitz again briefly. See what I mean? It's quite something! Take it easy with this one, though; just because it's full of goodness doesn't mean you won't pile on the pounds if you have too many.

Bircher Muesli

This is a fantastic way to start your day and will keep you going (almost) until lunchtime. You do have to be organized, as it needs to be made the night before. I tend to make a batch and divide it between several airtight glass jars. Kept in the fridge, it will last a few days. I've given quantities below, but they're just a guide. I tend to do it by eye and scale up or down, depending on how big a batch I want to make.

500g organic oats
1 litre cloudy apple juice
60g desiccated coconut
60g goji berries
60g pumpkin seeds
60g crushed walnuts (roughly break them up with your fingers before measuring)
2 tbsp chia seeds

Mix all the ingredients together in a large bowl before dividing between several small, airtight jars. Leave in the fridge overnight. In the morning you can either eat it as it is (I quite often grab a jar to eat later as I'm always running late), or, if you have time, add some blueberries and coconut yoghurt – delicious.

On a cold winter's morning, my breakfast of choice is porridge – and not just because I'm Scottish. I make mine with organic oats and almond milk, topped with a sliced banana, a sprinkling of ground cinnamon, a drizzle of honey and a scattering of seeds.

If I ever fancy toast for breakfast, I'll use rye bread and most likely top it with one of the following combinations:

- Almond butter, mashed avocado and sliced banana

- Poached egg with sliced avocado, fresh crab meat, spinach and tomato

- Poached egg with spinach and/or asparagus

I have these for lunch too, they work just as well.

Mid-morning snack

Three walnuts and a couple of Medjool dates or figs keep me going. A small cup of black coffee with a *tiny* dash of agave syrup to sweeten it, if I really need it. Sometimes my body craves a bit of sugar, but not always.

Lunch

If I'm on the hop and grabbing something light, then I'll have a bigger dinner to fill me up later. More often than not, though, I quite like having a big, late lunch so that I only have a little something to eat in the evening. One heavy meal a day is usually enough for me, otherwise I feel sluggish and bloated.

- Brown rice (about a quarter of one of those microwave packets) or half a take-away tub of Moroccan-style couscous with tuna (there's a tinned soy and ginger flavoured version by John West that I love) or salmon. Add a handful of spinach leaves, a few cherry tomatoes and some spicy baby beetroot. Mix it all up and *voilà*, a quick and easy lunch for one.

- A mushroom omelette with spinach and tomatoes on the side is super-quick and fills me up for a good few hours.

Nana's Special Soup

This is what my daughter, Amy, calls my mum's soup – she loves it! My granny used to make this for me when I was a child, and it makes me so happy to think that it's being passed down through the women in our family. Having said that, getting the recipe from my mum was tricky, as she's been making it so long she doesn't measure anything, so what follows below is a guide rather than a definitive recipe.

It's perfect if you're feeling under the weather, recovering from an operation or illness, or just want to fill up on hearty goodness. The lentils and barley are so good for you, it's ridiculous! They aren't just crammed with fibre, they're a source of phosphorus, selenium and manganese, which menopausal women need for the health of their bones, thyroid gland and hormone balance. They also contain vitamins B1 and B6, pantothenic acid, zinc and potassium.

a splash of vegetable oil
1 large white onion, peeled and roughly chopped

1 leek, washed, trimmed and sliced

3 large potatoes, peeled and cut into chunks

4–6 large carrots, topped, tailed, peeled and cut into chunks

2–4 skinless chicken breasts (you can use thighs instead, but if so, use 4–6)

1 litre chicken stock (you can swap this for miso if you'd like to add the health benefits of this fermented soy bean paste)

80g pearl barley, rinsed under the tap until the water runs clear

80g lentils, rinsed as above

salt and pepper, to season

Heat the vegetable oil in a large pot, add the onion and leek, and soften over a medium heat. Add the potatoes, carrots and the chicken, and cook for a minute or so until the chicken has whitened. Add the stock, pearl barley and lentils, stir well, season with salt and pepper, and bring to the boil. Reduce the heat and simmer for 15–20 minutes.

Scoop out half of the carrots and potatoes before they become too soft, and set aside in a bowl. The chicken should be cooked by now, too. Remove all of it from the pot, pull apart into smaller pieces and set aside in another bowl.

Return most of the potato and all the carrots to the pot. Use a hand blender to blitz into a smooth soup, then replace the remaining potato, along with the chicken. Season with more salt and pepper to taste.

······················· *Dinner* ·······················

I try to eat early. I like to be done and dusted by 7 p.m., so that my dinner has time to go down before bedtime. There's always the danger of in-front-of-telly snacking when you do this, so I try (I repeat 'try' – I don't always manage it) to make sure I don't end up nibbling the calorie equivalent of a second tea. Being tucked up in bed by 7.30 p.m. to avoid snacking would probably work too, but is a rather drastic option . . .

Dhal

This dish has all the wonderful goodness of lentils, plus the incredible taste of fresh spices. Like Nana's Special Soup, it tastes even better the following day. Don't be put off by the number of spices listed; once you have them in your cupboard they're easy to use, and last for ages.

It's worth noting that hot flushes can be triggered or exacerbated by what you eat, so while spicy food is great for boosting your metabolism, it can be less good for hormonal imbalance. If you're prone to flushes – and not all menopausal women are – then be careful with your spice intake and team the dish with a cooling yoghurt sauce. I have to stress, though, this isn't a hot dish by any means, so you won't break out in a sweat. It's just very, very tasty . . .

a splash of vegetable oil
1 tsp fennel seeds
1 tsp onion seeds
1 tsp cumin seeds
1 tsp brown mustard seeds

1 tsp chilli powder (or more if you prefer)
1 tsp paprika
1 tsp turmeric
2 white onions, finely chopped
4 garlic cloves, finely chopped
500g red lentils (soak these for 30 minutes beforehand,
*   preferably in filtered water, but tap water is OK)*
500ml water
1 x 400g tin chopped tomatoes
4cm piece fresh ginger, peeled and finely chopped or grated
2 bay leaves
1 tbsp coconut oil (more if you need it)
salt and pepper, to season

In a large pan, gently heat the oil and fry the seeds (*not* the ground spices) until they give off a lovely smell, then add the chilli powder, paprika, turmeric, onions and garlic, and stir over a moderate heat until soft.

Add the remaining ingredients, stir well again and bring to the boil. Reduce the heat, cover and simmer for at least an hour. Keep checking it, give it a little stir, and add water if it needs some. I like to let it sit for a few hours before serving, to allow the flavours to bed in.

Serve on its own in a bowl, or over brown rice if you really want to fill yourself up. You can also, as I mentioned earlier, team it with natural yoghurt. Some lime pickle garnished with fresh coriander and freshly squeezed lemon or lime juice is also a lovely side to this dish.

Miso soup. I'll have a bowl of this with fresh salmon, chilli, ginger, garlic, bok choi, broccoli, courgettes, sugar snap peas, and any other veg that I think will go. I don't cook anything separately, this is a one-pot dish – it all gets bunged in!

I simply add the miso paste and salmon to 500ml boiling water for a couple of minutes, throw in any other ingredients, simmer for a few minutes more and serve. I'll sometimes add dried noodles to the boiling water for the last 3 minutes if I need something a little more filling. It's such a quick and easy dish, and the miso paste is another good way of adding fermented food to your diet.

If you want to make this more like a ramen dish, don't add quite as much water to your bowl (so it's less of a soup), and top your noodles with a soft-boiled egg and some freshly torn coriander.

Chilli and ginger sea bass with broccoli. Finely chop a couple of centimetres of chilli, peel and grate a 10cm piece of ginger, and peel and finely chop one or two cloves of garlic. Fry over a medium heat in a splash of vegetable oil in a medium-sized pan, adding the sea bass skin-side down almost immediately. After a couple of minutes, gently turn the fish over then, after about another minute, remove it from the pan and set to one side. Add the broccoli to the hot pan and stir-fry in the remains of the chilli, garlic and ginger, with a splash of sesame oil.

As an alternative, sweep the sea bass through a mixture of flour, turmeric, salt and pepper before putting in the pan. You can also blanch the broccoli for 2 minutes in hot water to make it slightly less crunchy, if you like.

Salmon with sweet potato, coconut and chilli mash. Heat the oven to 180°C/350°F/gas mark 4 and bake the sweet potato, which can take 40 minutes to an hour, depending on its size.

Meanwhile, place a salmon steak on a sheet of tin foil with a finely chopped clove of garlic, a couple of centimetres of peeled and finely chopped ginger, some chopped fresh chilli (to taste, so however much you can take), a good squeeze of lemon juice, and a dash of salt and pepper. Gather the edges of the foil together and wrap to make a parcel. Transfer to a baking sheet and bake in the oven for 15 minutes.

Once cooked, allow to rest out of the oven for 2 minutes before serving. (If you prefer, you can pound the flavouring ingredients together in a pestle and mortar to make a paste to smear over the fish before sealing it in the foil.)

Once the sweet potato is baked, remove from the oven and allow to cool slightly. Cut in half and scoop out the flesh, then mash with some salt, pepper, a splash of coconut milk, some chopped chillies and the zest and juice of one lime. Delicious. (If baking a sweet potato takes too long for you, peel, cut the sweet potato into chunks and boil in water until soft. Drain and mash with salt, pepper and the juice of a squeezed orange – I add a splash of orange juice if I don't have any fresh fruit; it works just as well.)

Unwrap the salmon, place on top of the mash and serve with salad.

Snack while watching telly

Hummus and wholemeal pitta or thin crackers. The tasty chickpea dip contains vitamins K and B6, phosphorus, folate, zinc and copper, and is a good source of protein and fibre.

Microwave popcorn. OK, it's not as super-healthy if you eat the sweet 'n' salty flavour (my favourite), but it's a good source of fibre and relatively low in calories. You could even try it plain – it's better than you think!

A cheeky glass of wine. I'm a big believer that unless you need to abstain for health reasons, telling yourself that you can never have something again is a sure-fire way to want nothing else. Just knowing I can have a glass if I want to, but remembering that I'll feel better if I don't have it simply out of habit, means I can take it or leave it. And that way I enjoy it more when I do settle down to a Netflix binge with a chilled glass by my side!

By making changes to your diet, you can ease a lot of the discomfort the menopause throws at you. A better diet is better for you anyway, as your body ages. You can boil it down to some simple bullet points as I've done, and you'll see that there's absolutely nothing new here – you just have to commit to making it happen:

• Make sure you have plenty of calcium in your diet: milk, yoghurt, kale, tinned fish complete with the bones.

• Eat less junk – your body is going through a tough time, so give it the nourishment it needs. You'll feel better for it.

• Drink lots of water – it's not only good for the body but it also helps your skin stay plump and hydrated, too.

• Drink less alcohol, especially in the evenings, when the sugar slips through your lips and lands on your hips, and you're not moving from in front of the telly to work it off.

• Stay clear of spicy foods in the evening too, especially if you're suffering with night sweats – they only make things worse.

- No caffeine after lunch – it only adds to the sleepless tossing and turning.

That doesn't sound like a whole lot of fun but believe me, when you start to feel better you'll be wolfing down the bok choi!

I think the key thing to remember is that you are *not* going on a diet. Changing what you eat in order to make your menopausal symptoms easier to contend with shouldn't feel like a punishment, which, to me, most diets in the traditional, weight-loss sense do. What you're doing is making a lifestyle change that will become a natural part of your everyday routine, and in many ways will add new and exciting dishes to your day rather than removing them.

Health through food is the most natural thing in the world. It's only because we've become so accustomed to eating in a certain way – from the first tuna pasta we ever made when we left home, through to the kids' tea and partner's dinner – that we've forgotten how to eat for *us,* in a way that suits *our* bodies. Let this be just one of the good changes the menopause brings.

Dr Peers Says . . .

DIET AND THE MENOPAUSE

We should all be eating a healthy, varied diet, based on starchy foods and plenty of fruit and vegetables, and low in saturated fat, sugar and salt, regardless of our life stage. However, during and after the menopause, women need to pay particular attention to maintaining a diet that not only reduces the risk of developing cardiovascular disease and osteoporosis but also helps with the day-to-day menopausal symptoms caused by declining levels of oestrogen.

Women can lose up to 20 per cent of their bone density in the five to seven years after the menopause. The body can't produce its own calcium and relies on the foods we eat for daily supplies. When we don't get enough calcium in our diet, the body takes it from the bones, making them weaker and prone to breakage. Therefore, making sure we have enough calcium is important for the maintenance of bone strength and density, and prevention of osteoporosis.

• The recommended daily intake of calcium is 700mg for adults and this can generally be achieved by ensuring that calcium-rich foods, such as dairy products and leafy green vegetables, are included in the diet.

• Focusing on calcium alone is not enough; we also need to make sure we have sufficient vitamin D. It helps the body to absorb the calcium and contributes to muscle strength. In the summer months, this can be achieved by eating foods such as oily fish, eggs, red meat and fortified foods, plus a short daily walk in the sunshine. In the darker days of autumn and winter, we need a little help and a daily supplement (1000μg vitamin D3) is recommended. It's advisable to have your vitamin D levels checked by your GP. A very high percentage of my patients are deficient in vitamin D as we have very little sun exposure in the winter months and we all use cosmetics and creams with an SPF to protect our skin from sun damage.

• Women who are postmenopausal have a greater risk of developing cardiovascular disease, therefore a heart-healthy diet is particularly important. This involves:

– Helping to reduce your cholesterol levels by minimizing the amount of saturated fat – swap butter and coconut oil for rapeseed, olive and sunflower oils and spreads.

– Eating oily fish (such as mackerel, salmon or sardines) twice a week.

– Helping your blood pressure by keeping your salt intake below 6g a day.

– Lower your risk of heart disease, stroke and some cancers by eating your five fruits and vegetables a day.

– Keep your digestive system healthy by including lots of fibre in your diet, for example, wholegrain breakfast cereals, wholewheat pasta and pulses.

– Limiting your alcohol consumption to no more than 14 units a week and making sure you have several alcohol-free days.

• Women post-menopause are prone to metabolic syndrome, where the body doesn't respond as it should to insulin production and thus very high levels of insulin are produced by the pancreas. This causes an increase in weight, especially in the midriff, and can also increase your blood pressure, cholesterol and risk of heart disease. Exercise and a diet containing foods with a low glycaemic index (GI), together with HRT, can really help.[1]

1 *Sources: British Nutrition Foundation. www.nutrition.org.uk/healthyliving/lifestages/menopause.html; NHS UK. Women's Health 40–60. www.nhsuk.com/LiveWell; National Osteoporosis Foundation. Nutrition. www.nof.org/patients/*

8

Keep on Moving

....

'Swimming works for me (ten years in). Concentrate on nothing but breathing. Lovely to clear the brain fog and you don't notice the hot flushes.'

'We need to keep active with weight-bearing exercises to maintain bone health. Resistance training is also good to build muscle as our muscle mass decreases with age.'

'Running! I find it clears my head, helps me to refocus and also helps with my aches and pains in some bizarre way!'

'Long walks with a good friend take my mind off it for a while . . .'

....

Fighting the middle jiggle

There's a reason it's called 'middle-age spread'. It's because it bloody well is. I have one failsafe way to know when it's time to lay off the crisps and do some sit-ups: I simply drive down my road. If as soon as I hit the bumpy bit my middle begins to jiggle, then I *know*. I've tried not to be bothered about it, and shrug and say, 'Meh, this is just how I am now', but then I drive down that damn road again, get the middle jiggle and I think, 'Nope. I am *not* ready to give in just yet.'

The difference between thinking that and doing something about it is even more daunting now, because during the menopause we're effectively running to stand still. Not that I run – I hate running – but it's likely that all the things you used to do to keep trim just won't seem to be enough to keep on top of things any more.

REM may well have been talking about menopausal women when they sang that 'Everybody hurts ...' I don't know a single woman going through the menopause who doesn't let out a mighty *ooof!* every time she stands up or sits down, me included. My neck hurts, my back hurts, my knees hurt. Sometimes, I swear, my *hair* hurts.

What can you do about it? I try to stay active because if you sit about for too long, there's a real possibility that you'll never move again. And just think how bored you'd get, stuck in the one place for the rest of your life. So keep moving, find your own pace, then push it up a notch ... That's when you'll begin to see and feel the difference.

Exercise is good for you. We all know that. We all know how important it is to have a healthy diet *and* an active lifestyle – and not just because of the effect the two things have on how we look on the outside. It's truer than ever when you're menopausal, with recent studies suggesting that exercise could be a natural alternative to HRT because of the impact it has on our mental health as well as on our bodies.

Feeling good in body and brain

Feeling good about yourself physically goes a long way to helping you out mentally; the two go hand in hand. I *like* feeling fit and strong, and keeping my body active makes my mind work better too. I get bored easily, though, so I either have to find a gym buddy (who isn't going to get on my nerves by being overly enthusiastic) or a trainer that I like.

Most of us who are of menopausal age will have 'felt the burn' in the gym at one time or another and not in a hot flush kind of way, for once! Aerobics, aqua, spinning, Zumba – all of these classes are brilliant for burning calories and working your muscles. However, none of them has ever floated my boat, mainly because they involve thrashing about and getting very, very sweaty, but also because I'm useless at exercise classes. I get confused between left and right, and always end up bumping into people, which makes them cross and me embarrassed.

I've never been to a Zumba class, but I hear they're wonderful. I just know I'd be too self-conscious to fling myself around with the abandon that would be expected of me. I did buy a Zumba DVD once, but following one attempt after I'd put the kids to bed, when I banged my hip on the kitchen unit and couldn't keep up with the perky and irritatingly enthusiastic woman in micro shorts, I put down my maracas (yes, I even bought the maracas to jolly things up a little . . .), poured myself a glass of wine and never did it again. Does that sound familiar?

I've learned that I like doing exercise alone, so that's why going to the gym and stuffing earphones in works for me. I don't listen to pumping tunes or anything like that; it's usually

Woman's Hour, a TED Talk or a podcast. I like to listen to people talking, and think about what they're saying as I'm lifting weights. It makes the time go by faster, and it's nice to think that I'm learning something while I'm working out.

Keeping fit isn't just about getting a tight bum, in my opinion. It's common sense that moving our bodies, and shaking off the lethargy we all suffer from increasingly as we age, is going to make us feel better. To a greater or lesser degree, we use fitness to make ourselves feel better every day – that walk for a bit of fresh air, the stretch after you've been hunched over a computer for hours, the trot round the block to blow the cobwebs away. We *know* we feel better after moving, even on a low level.

What's more, when it comes to anxiety, depression and stress, all of which are associated with the menopause, it has been *proven* that the endorphins our body releases when we exercise go a long way to making us feel better; about ourselves *and* the situation we're in. We can think more clearly, grey clouds lift, and our energy levels rise, which of course makes us feel more able to face the troubles in our mind.

Over the years, I've spoken to many celebrities who've told me that the reason they exercise is not for the six-pack or the enviably sculpted arms, but to clear the fog in their head and give them the energy they need to confront whatever difficulties they might be up against. I've mentioned before about how important our mental health is when it comes to coping with everything the menopause throws at us, but many of us forget that we can work our bodies to help ourselves mentally. For a woman who loves to multitask, there's no better reason than that to get up, get out, and shake it all about . . .

Weight training

You may have flirted with exercise in the past, but the years of the menopause is a time when you really need it, and your body will thank you for making the effort. The notion of exercising to build strength and stamina rather than change how you look might be difficult to get your head around because, let's face it, for most of our lives we've forced ourselves to do sit-ups because our tummies jiggle and not because we're thinking about building our muscles. While looking more toned is an obvious side effect (and a welcome one!), in this instance it isn't so much to do with how you look, but everything to do with what it will do for your health, and how it will make your body feel.

If you've never tried it before, this may sound odd to you, but I enjoy weight training. It's slow and steady. It's all about refined moves, and you can work at your own pace, all the while getting stronger and stronger without bulking up, which is what women usually worry about when it comes to weights. It doesn't make you sweat too much, which is inevitable with cardiovascular training, and there's little chance of falling over. Which is good news when you're as clumsy as I am.

Aerobic exercise is essential for good health but it's only part of the picture, so thank God weight lifting is the new running for the over-forties! In order to prevent the dreaded spread, and to firm up, strength training is the key.

I know what you're thinking: weight lifting is for gym bunnies, posers, or for men with too much testosterone. I hear you! They are just some of the many reasons women hate going to the gym. Weight lifting, however, is great. Hear me out. You don't have to start lugging huge barbells around, or pouting and taking selfies, and you won't end up ripped like a body builder. Well, clearly you will if you really put the time and effort in, but that's not the level of fitness or dedication I'm talking about. I mean building up enough muscle to keep you strong.

Even Sheila Hancock, the beautiful octogenarian actress, has said that at the age of eighty-four she became a weight-lifting convert, after suffering from muscle wastage in her arms. She had apparently begun to find it difficult to lift her luggage into the overhead compartments on aeroplanes – something I struggle with and I'm thirty-seven years younger than her! She decided to do something about it, and weight training was the answer. One of the things I loved most about the *Daily Mail* article where she revealed this new regime was when she said, 'Some people do weights to look toned but I just want to stay strong as I get older. You don't have to get weak as you get older – I've proved that.' Go, Sheila!

I know what she means. It's so disheartening when you can't lift your own bag higher than your head, and it's so thrilling when you eventually can. I'm personally relieved that weight training has been shown to be one of the most beneficial exercises for menopausal women in terms of building crucial muscle mass, developing strength and improving balance, because it's something that you can do *sloooowly* and carefully, while still feeling great afterwards.

To me it makes sense to combine strength training with stretching exercises, so that muscles and tendons become strong and also flexible. I'm not the world's most flexible person, and the day I'm able to touch my toes while keeping my legs straight might never come. However, stretching in other ways stops my back from seizing up and my neck from going into complete spasm – which it seems to enjoy doing – so anything that takes that pain away is worth looking into.

As we all lose muscle mass as we age – men as well as women – it's important to do some kind of strength training to build them up again. It will also help your body stay strong against osteoporosis, osteoarthritis and type 2 diabetes. You don't have to lift crazily heavy weights to get the benefits and if you don't like the idea of going to a gym, invest in a few weights for yourself and try some of the following exercises at home – I do most of my workouts in my bedroom, in my pyjamas!

Waist-toning twists. To combat a thickening or wobbly waist, hold a weight against your chest with both hands. I started off using a 5kg dumbbell and built up to a 10kg weight over time, but select whichever weight you can handle but takes some effort. If it's too easy then you won't get the same benefit, so you may as well push yourself!

Place your feet shoulder-width apart, then twist your upper body from side to side 20 times to complete 1 set. Do this for a further 2 sets (i.e. 3 sets of 20 reps in total). In between sets, I take the weight in one hand, drop my arm down by my side, hold my stomach in, and lean over to the side that is holding the weight. Come back up again and repeat 10 times, before swapping hands and doing the other side.

21s – bicep curls. Holding a 5kg dumbbell in each hand, stand with your feet shoulder-width apart. Start with your arms down by your sides, palms facing forwards. For 7 reps, lift both weights together, bending at the elbow, until your forearms are parallel to the ground. Then, starting with your forearms parallel to the ground, palms facing upwards, bend your arms at the elbow, lifting the weights up to shoulder height for another 7 reps. Finally, bring your arms back down to your sides, palms facing forwards again, and this time lift the weights all the way to shoulder height – bending at the elbows again – 7 times. You'll have done 21 reps in total now – that's why it's called 21s!

If you're concerned about straining your back, start with lighter weights, and *always* hold your stomach in and hoist your pelvic floor up before you start lifting. This keeps the muscles around your core active, so they act like a girdle, protecting you from injury.

Squats. We all know what squats are. They look ungainly and Instagram seems to be filled with pert-bottomed women sticking their bums out whilst holding impossibly heavy weights. But if you can't beat them, join them. Squats are good for you, as they work the largest muscle group in your body (your butt and legs), and burn a crazy number of calories. That's why they're harder than they look; you're doing so much!

Stand with your feet just wider than shoulder-width apart. Hold a 10kg dumbbell with both hands and, keeping your arms straight, let it hang down between your legs. Try to keep your back upright as you squat down so that the dumbbell almost touches the floor, before bringing yourself back up to standing. Do 3 sets of 10 reps – your bottom will thank you! Allow the dumbbell to hang, as you aren't exercising your arms here, you're just using the weight for extra *oomph*.

When time is of the essence
• **Bicep curls.** We all need to go to the loo a few times a day and if your pelvic floor ain't what it used to be, then you could

be going more than ever! To maximize your time spent in the bathroom, my sister told me to try this: she leaves a pair of weights in there, one on either side of the loo. So, each time she sits down, she grabs the weights and does a few reps, either bringing her arms above her head, out to the side, or up to her shoulders in bicep curls. Who knew you could be toning up while spending a penny?

• **Squats.** Do you have an electric toothbrush? Most of us do nowadays, and they usually come with a buzzer to tell us when we've brushed our teeth for long enough. That's about 2 minutes. So, every time you brush your teeth, squat. Right there in the bathroom. You get can about twenty out in that time. That's forty a day. That's 280 a week. That's 1,120 a month. Who says you don't have time to exercise? If squatting gets boring, do some lunges. Or squat into a chair position against your bathroom wall while you brush your teeth. Your bum and thigh muscles will scream at you while you do it, but you won't half feel the benefit!

• **Pelvic floor.** *Always remember your 'one-twos'.* I've put that in bold because it's really important. Whenever you can, wherever you are, whatever you're doing, do your one-twos. This is to exercise your pelvic floor muscles and it will strengthen you from the inside out when you exercise. It will help improve your core strength and stability, you'll be less worried about peeing yourself when you sneeze, and your sex life will improve as well, as you'll be improving the blood supply to the area, increasing nerve activity and as those muscles become stronger so too will your orgasms. Pretty amazing, eh? All you need to do is think of how it feels to hold in a fart, or a number one and a number two, all at the same time. We've all done it, don't be shy. Squeeze your nunny and your bum, and engage your stomach muscles before doing any exercise.

I could say that's all there is to it, but there is of course a lot more going on than you'd think. Essentially, this is what you have to remember – *one-two*! I personally find that if I start thinking about the pelvic floor, holding for 10 seconds and breathing and releasing and imagining a lift going up and down (which is the line you may have heard in yoga or Pilates), I get bored and I won't do it. But thinking about one-two, hold in a wee and a poo! Yup, I can remember that. Give it a go, whenever it pops into your head. Do it right now as you're reading this. See, it works, doesn't it?

The 7-minute workout
There are lots of 7-minute workout apps out there to choose from, and you can pick a level that suits you. They're all pretty similar, though, and built around the principle of high-intensity interval training, using your own bodyweight as resistance. So perhaps you'll exercise for 30 seconds, then rest for 10, then go again. The beauty of these workouts is that you can do them anywhere – in a living room, an office, a park.

My mum has even started doing them. She's seventy-two and has been feeling a bit out of sorts recently as she stopped smoking a year ago and has put on a little weight around the middle. Now, she still looks fantastic, but she doesn't like how it's making her feel (something we can all relate to) and she doesn't feel comfortable joining an aerobics class with lots of intimidatingly fit ladies. So she's started doing these workouts at home and the last time we spoke (she lives round the corner, so we speak all the time) she was just starting to turn a corner and feel a bit like her old self again. Or her slightly younger, stronger self. You know what I mean.

Fitness after a hysterectomy

As well as strength training, the benefits of aerobic exercise, such as walking, are well known, and walking is an activity that's even more important during the menopause as it can combat mood changes and weight gain. A brisk or even medium-paced walk is really good for you. It'll boost your energy, build muscle and make you smile. Walking is *always* recommended as a form of exercise, particularly when you're getting back to fitness after a hysterectomy.

There were two things I did to get fit after my operation. The first involved setting myself a challenge. And the second was a challenge that was set for me . . .

Walking with purpose

A month or so after coming out of hospital I felt ready to start pushing myself physically, but as much as I need a reason to do it (being well and feeling like myself again is a pretty good reason), I also need a goal. At the time, my teenage son, Fin, had signed up to do his Duke of Edinburgh's Award. Part of that involved a physical challenge, so he was gearing up for his first ever hiking experience.

I was really proud of him but I also thought, 'What can I do as a mum that would motivate him? To show him that even if things get difficult, it doesn't mean we should shirk our commitment to something – it means we should get our heads down and push through it!' So I looked into doing a challenge of my own. That year was the diamond anniversary of the Duke of Edinburgh's Award, which meant that anyone could set themselves a one-off challenge. I decided that I'd like to do a marathon.

Now let me quickly add that I intended to walk it – I've told you, I am *not* a runner. I've done quite a few walking marathons for charity in the past – both full and half – so I knew I'd be able to do it with enough training. So Nick and I started by doing a few gentle walks to see how I felt. The first one finished when I got to the end of my street. I was shaking and dizzy, hanging on to Nick for support.

It became very clear after the first few attempts, as we pushed the distance up, that I was in *no way* capable of walking a marathon two months after my operation. So we sensibly cut it down to a half-marathon, and sent off our application. Finding a day when we could both do the walk was difficult, but the timing was entirely up to us and so the week in between Christmas and New Year seemed like a sensible option. I had some time off work so I could rest, both before and after.

Christmas Eve arrived and we did what we always do: we took the whole family – all the kids and my parents – to see a panto, everyone in their Christmas jumpers. Afterwards, we went for a meal, and that's when disaster struck: I ate some food that had dairy in it. I'm severely lactose intolerant, which is not a fad, or a diet choice, or a whim; it's a full-on intolerance. After a few mouthfuls I realized I could taste the familiar coating on the roof of my mouth and checked with the waiter. Yes, the dish had both cream *and* soft cheese in it. Gulp.

I drank as much water as I could to try to flush the dairy

out of my system, but it was no use. By the time we got home my stomach was so bloated I looked seven months pregnant. An hour later I was on the loo, and I then spent the rest of the night throwing up . . . all the way into Christmas Day, which I spent in bed with a raging migraine, curtains drawn and retching. Not the best of times . . .

Three days later and I thought I felt well enough to try the walk. So Nick and I laced up our trainers, pulled on our bobble hats and headed into London. I wanted to start at Buckingham Palace, as our walk was for a royal charity. We logged our route, flagged up our Just Giving page and headed off. Four miles in and we found ourselves squashed up against a billion tourists at Tower Bridge. I had a serious sense-of-humour failure and wanted to push them all into the Thames. Nick stayed calm, which infuriated me even more, so I stalked off (OK, I walked one foot ahead of him, squished between lost people with cameras who had *clearly* never used a pavement before and found the whole process of *moving forward* too taxing!).

When it quietened down a little, we found a stall that sold the best coffee in the world. This is a fact, because they sold coffee with *alcohol* in it, and boy did I need it. Doing this walk had been an *incredibly stupid* idea, and I was *very grumpy* about it. I didn't want to quit because once I say I'm going to do something I follow through, even if it's a really bad idea. So I was stuck with it.

Nick and I walked the next few miles in silence. Then I needed a wee, so we found a pub that wasn't too full of drunk people and moved on again. By now my bad mood had evaporated (the restorative powers of walking in action), and I squeezed Nick's hand and told him I was sorry for being such a mardy arse. He hugged me and said it was OK, which made me feel awful.

By Mile 10, my feet hurt, my legs hurt and my face was so cold I could barely move it. By Mile 12 my surgery scars were throbbing, and we were once again walking in silence; a determined one this time. By now we had done a loop, and had worked out that by just over Mile 13 we would be at Clapham Junction, from where we could catch a train home. So we headed to the station, just the two of us, in the dark and cold. When we arrived we checked our miles and made sure we'd completed our half-marathon. We had: 13.32 miles – 27,400 steps – in just under four hours. I was *knackered*. We high-fived each other, had a hug, then got on the train home. As soon as we got home I crawled into a hot bath and lay in it until I was wrinkly. Every part of me hurt.

As I sat downstairs later that evening, wrapped in my pyjamas, socks and fluffy dressing gown, and cradling a lovely glass of wine, Nick and I checked our Just Giving page. We'd managed to raise over £600 for charity. It felt good. Not only had I set myself a goal and achieved it (OK, I'd not done it with the best attitude; there had been a slight huffiness part-way through . . .) but I'd also raised some money for an incredible cause. We weren't talking Live Aid sums exactly, but every little helps, and I'm glad I did my bit.

Have I done anything else like it since then? Have I heck! I lost my big toenail on one foot afterwards, so that put paid to any more long-distance walking. I've carried on going to the gym, doing yoga, and swimming; mixing things up so that when one gets dull I do one of the others. Whatever you do, the key is to keep on moving.

My body story

I said there were two things I did to get fit after my operation. The half marathon was a personal thing, which I did for my own sense of achievement, to raise money for charity and to set a good example for my son. The second thing was an equally worthy cause – *Loose Women*'s Body Stories campaign – but was rather more of an incentive to get fit. Just a couple of months after the half-marathon I'd be standing in my pants in front of my teenage heartthrob, Bryan Adams.

Loose Women had asked him to take and release an untouched photo for a campaign we were launching with the hashtag #MyBodyMyStory, and because he's a lovely man, he thought it was a great idea and agreed to do it. So, one February afternoon I, and eight other Loose Women, walked barefoot into a brightly lit glass-walled room and let our bathrobes fall to the floor. We stood in all our glory, women aged from twenty-seven to seventy, our bodies swathed in life's badges of honour: stretch marks, cellulite, broken veins, caesarean and hysterectomy scars, age spots, wobbly bits and firm bits – they were all on display. The photograph went on to make headlines around the world as a celebration of women, flaws and all!

Finding your own reason to get fit and healthy is the only way to make you stick at it. Whether it's for health reasons that mean you don't have the choice, for personal reasons where you need a goal to motivate you or, in my case, both of these things – with the added pressure of the *Loose Women* team coming up with the ingenious idea of having us all stand in our underwear for the whole world to see! There are plenty of fitness options to choose from – what's yours?

Swimming

Swimming was recommended to me by a friend of mine as a way of using exercise to clear the mind. She'd experienced intense anxiety after a serious, life-threatening illness and told me she used to get to the pool early in the morning and swim up and down, up and down, focusing on her breathing and her stroke. Breathe and stroke. Breathe and stroke. After a while, she said, her anxiety would fade away, and all that mattered was doing the perfect front crawl.

As well as helping with your mental health, studies have shown that swimming (along with walking or jogging) can make you less prone to hot flushes and painful joints during the menopause. It's going to help with your weight, too, of course. What really enticed me into getting back in the water was the prospect of all the stuff that whirrs around your head when you're in the full throes of the menopause just fading away for a while – the sadness, the lack of motivation, the aggression, the stress. Sounds good, doesn't it?

A few days after speaking to my friend, I decided to give it a go. I used to swim as a teen and also during my pregnancies, but I hadn't done it for quite a while. I turned up at the pool early one winter's morning along with all the elderly members of the gym, waiting for it to open. I had *never* been there so early before! I got changed, shivering as my bare feet hit the cold floor, and padded over to the pool. There was just me and a few older gentlemen that first morning, slowly making our way up and down, up and down.

Once the shock of being in the water wore off, I understood what my friend had been talking about. As my heart pounded, my racing mind slowed. I'd forgotten how intense swimming is, and how hard it is! If you can sweat underwater, that's exactly what I was doing. I was out of breath, my heart was nearly bursting out of my chest, and my arms really hurt. I'd thought I was fit!

I've continued to swim at least once a week, and I still enjoy it. It's quicker than going to the gym as fifteen minutes of going up and down is enough to get my heart pounding, but if I have the time and inclination I do more. I like that once I'm in the water no one can see me, or judge me. It's not about keeping up with anyone else, or wearing the right gear, it's simply about moving forward. It doesn't cost the earth – most of us have a local pool we can use, without being a gym member. I feel refreshed and ready to face the day once I've had my swim; who wouldn't want to feel that?

Yoga

Yoga is a great way to improve your flexibility, but it's not all about being a Bendy Wendy. Learning how to control your breathing while you work through a series of poses is a wonderful way to help combat stress. Practising yoga is also widely known to help ease symptoms of the menopause – it can improve sleep, heighten your mood and reduce pain by giving your muscles a much-needed stretch.

I don't go to any classes but instead choose to use an app called Asana Rebel, which I like because it's on my phone and I can use it anywhere: in my bedroom wearing my pyjamas, in my dressing room at work, or in a hotel room if I'm on the road. If I can only fit in a quick five minutes, then that's all I do. If I have more time to spare, then I'll do the half-hour workout and really get some heat going.

You might not think that doing yoga can get your heart pounding, but it can! There are times when I hate it, and

I bitch and moan all the way through, grumbling to myself as there's no one there forcing me to plaster an 'I'm really enjoying this' look on my face. I might not always like it at the time, but I sure as hell like how I feel afterwards. My middle feels like it's pulled in, my back feels stronger and my thighs, once they've stopped shaking, feel tighter. And on the days when I'm really enjoying it, it's wonderful. I feel strong, supple and clear-headed as I breathe deeply in and out during each move. It's lovely.

Fitness in menopause is all about finding what works for *you*. So be realistic. If you're struggling to get started, set yourself goals that are attainable. Saying 'I'm going to run' isn't going to cut it – the best way to do it is to be incremental and specific. Why not say, 'I'm going to run for 10 minutes, three times a week'. Then you can up it when you feel ready. If you don't enjoy it, then try something else!

You don't have to join in with the latest craze either. Let's face it, we probably did it all the first time around, from inline skating to body pump. Although, I *am* considering trying boxercise . . . It looks like uncoordinated dancing with cartoon gloves on, whacking a bag to get rid of pent-up frustration and aggression. And if there's anyone who needs to get rid of suppressed rage, it's a menopausal woman!

Dr Peers Says . . .

MENOPAUSAL MUSCLE LOSS

Although weight gain may not be directly linked to the menopause, changes in fat distribution and in the proportion of muscle mass and body fat happen as women age. There's a transition from fat deposits below the waist (the pear-shaped body) to deposits above the waist (apple-shaped body) as well as a gradual decrease in muscle mass (which burns more calories) and an increase in body fat (which burns fewer calories). All this means the number of calories the body needs each day is reduced.

Oestrogen is important for the production of elastin and collagen in the muscles, as is testosterone. A decrease in these hormones after the menopause will result in thinning of the muscles and less stamina for exercise. HRT and testosterone replacement can restore muscle health, improve muscle definition and thus improve a woman's body confidence and shape.[1]

DON'T STOP MOVING . . .

Being physically active during the menopause has many benefits. It can contribute to bone health by promoting the movement of calcium into your bones. It can also reduce the risk of cardiovascular disease and, although not proven, there's evidence that a solid exercise regime can relieve stress and enhance quality of life. It can also help with the frequency and severity of hot flushes as it increases the levels of beta-endorphins (chemicals released in response to pain, stress and trauma) in the brain, and helps improve sleep and relieve depression.

Regular, gentle exercise that works your heart a little (aerobic) and increases bone density (weight-bearing) is the best approach. Weight-bearing exercises are those that involve moving your body against gravity and they can be either low or high impact. Running, aerobics, racquet sports (such as tennis), dancing and stair climbing are all high impact. Exercises such as brisk walking or stair-step machines are low-impact exercises.

Muscle-strengthening exercises, such as the use of weights or resistance bands, are also important. When your muscles pull on your bones, they boost bone strength.[2]

1 *Sources: Weight Watchers UK. www.weightwatchers.co.uk; North American Menopause Society. www.menopause.org*

2 *Sources: Women's Health Concern. Osteoporosis: Bone health following the menopause. www.womens-health-concern.org; Menopause Health Matters. Exercise for women in the menopause. www.menopausehealth-matters.com; National Osteoporosis Foundation. Exercise to stay healthy. www.nof.org/patients; Menopause and your bone strength. NHS Live Well. www.nhs.uk*

9

Through the Menopause – and Beyond

There are lots of reasons why I'm passionate about writing about the menopause. Top of the list is because I'm experiencing it myself, so I'm naturally interested in it. However, I experience lots of things that I don't feel the burning *need* to get down on the page and share with other women. The main reason for my passion is because *nobody wants to talk about it*.

Now, I understand why no one wants to be associated with something society has, somewhere down the line, decided makes you officially old, knackered, past it, useless and pretty much a laughing stock. Who would want to throw their hat into that ring? But why *does* a society that has changed so much in the past decade – with men and women living longer, healthier and more productive lives than at any other time in our history – still use the menopause as a barometer to measure a woman's usefulness and status in society?

We aren't cavemen any more! We aren't just here to procreate, carry on the race and then pop off. We haven't been so black and white in our thinking for hundreds of years, so why are women still viewed in a certain way once they reach a certain age? The only way that the menopausal years can be accepted as a normal part of life for half of the world's population is if we change society's perception of it.

Thankfully, things do appear to be changing, and one of the ways we can continue to move forward is to educate *all* women (including younger women, so they can be aware of what to expect – especially as the menopause can strike early) to ensure they know what's out there in terms of medication, how they can look after their physical and mental health, and generally how to feel the best they possibly can. Think about it: women now are living into their eighties and nineties. The menopause starts making an impact on a woman's body in her forties and generally comes to the fore in her fifties. Do you *really* want to spend so much of your life feeling dreadful?

It's also crucially important to educate men. Women don't exist in a bubble of womanhood; we have partners, sons, fathers and brothers whom we love and live with. If we have no idea how to cope with the changes our minds and bodies are going through, then it stands to reason that they won't be too clued-up on how to deal with them either. You might feel uncomfortable bringing up the subject, and it might not be an easy conversation to have, but it will help massively in the long run.

Keep it light-hearted, if you prefer, but let the men in your life know what you're going through, and explain why. You know the science behind it now, as you've almost finished this book. In fact, give them this book! Through open conversation a circle of understanding will spiral outwards: the men in our lives might work with women who may be experiencing the menopause, perhaps, and will be more inclined to behave in a more sympathetic and understanding fashion. We'll have indirectly helped women outside our own homes, women we don't even know, and at some point menopause won't be perceived as anything untoward, it will just be another talking point – like puberty and pregnancy – and will be addressed with the same lack of embarrassment.

Hello, I'm still here!

One of the most pressing issues surrounding the menopause, beyond the physical symptoms but wrapped up with the mental impact it has on women, is the feeling of invisibility that comes with ageing. Genetically speaking, we're programmed to be attracted to the younger, vibrant and healthy members of the species, purely from the point of view of procreation and the continuation of the human race. However, as intelligent beings, surely we should have moved on from that. The elders of the tribe should be treated with dignity and respect, not tossed aside like food past its sell-by date.

How do I feel about being middle-aged? Pretty much the same as you do, I'd imagine. It's been a strange thing to get my head around. It sneaks up on you, I guess. One day you're one of the young ones at work, with your bright eyes, shiny face and endless enthusiasm, and the next you're gulping in shock when some bushy-tailed youngster tells you that they'd love to be as smart as/as funny as/look as good as you when they're your age.

Suddenly, those three words – 'for your age' – start creeping into every conversation. *You look good for your age. Aren't you trendy for your age? Aren't you fast for your age?* A phrase you had considered problematic, and had probably unwittingly used yourself, is being thrown right back atcha, and it's your turn to suck it up.

I'm just entering middle age and I have no intention of doing so in the spirit of defeat. I've just started to figure myself out – I know what I like and don't like, what I'm going to spend my time on and what I'm definitely not going to waste it doing. I'm more creative than I've ever been because I have the experience to know what works and what doesn't. I feel relevant to my peers – and that's what matters.

I don't want to compete with twenty-year-olds. They're just starting out on their journey. I know I'm way ahead of them in terms of experience, and I'm aware that I'm probably falling behind in terms of relevance, at least in their eyes. However, I now feel that I am what I am, and that's OK. I'm me. I hope you feel the same – that you're happy in your own skin.

In fact, I don't think there's ever been a better time to be middle-aged; older women are smashing through barriers and boundaries in beauty, fashion, business and media. We're surrounded by women who are coming into their own as they enter their middle years, showing that anything is possible, and to me they are examples of a life well lived, filled with experiences that they're ready to call on during the second half of it. What they're not ready to do is slope off and be forgotten about.

In any case, once you get to the top of the hill, who's to say that means you're over it? What if the top of the hill is a beautiful plateau, where all the lessons you learned during the ascent can be put to fantastic use? It's not often you'll hear a middle-aged woman quote Miley Cyrus and her alter ego, Hannah Montana, as a point of heroic reference, but listen to the words of her song 'The Climb'. It'll get you, I know it will, because to paraphrase Miley, it really isn't about how fast you get to the top, or what's waiting on the other side, it's all about the climb.

Life really is all about the journey. It's the only one we've got, and everything that we do today to make our lives better has a bearing on how our tomorrows will be. When it comes to our own health and happiness, we have to take responsibility for both of those things by doing something positive about them before it's too late.

What on earth to wear

So, we know how much stuff there is going on physically and mentally during the menopause, and we've talked a lot about what's happening to your body and how you can help to look after yourself. Unless you're incredibly self-confident and robust, your appearance will naturally affect the way you feel about yourself.

The way I see it, the changes that we're going through on the inside can mark a change for the good on the outside. I know it's a challenge when your metabolism is slowing down and your waist is thickening, but all is not lost. I also know that I dress differently now to how I did ten years ago, but the main reason behind that is not my body shape, it's because I now dress for *myself*. I'm not trying to keep up with fashion, or what I think I should be wearing. I wear what I like! It is, without doubt, one of the major perks of growing older.

Funnily enough, if there's one thing over the past few years that people have noticed about me, it's the change in my dress sense. Ever since I stopped wearing what I thought I should, I've taken more risks, and, bizarrely, I probably now dress in a younger fashion style than I used to, just because I like it. Granted, it's my version of things – I'm never going to fit into the same slinky little outfit that a twenty-something would, but I can still push the boat out from time to time.

Having said that, I certainly dress for comfort a lot more, rather than slobbing around in my old maternity trousers (yes, I held on to them for almost fifteen years, because a) they were comfy, and b) I liked that they were a little bit baggy, so I felt slim in them. Don't judge me!). I now own some comfortable clothes that actually look *good*. I've stopped having a 'presentable to the outside world' wardrobe that involved wearing Spanx and tight shoes, and 'clothes that should be burned and buried in a lead box' while at home. Spanx and heels are now purely for a 'do', and the rest of the time I wear soft jumpers, stretchy jeans and fashion trainers. My feet and my internal organs are thankful for the extra space, and I feel good about myself!

I can't stress enough that this has nothing to do with dressing 'younger' and trying to deny the age you are. It's most definitely about being comfortable in your own skin, and I think fashion has reached a point where we can now wear pretty much what we like, whatever our age. Nothing makes an outfit look as good as one that is worn with confidence. So, I say, if you like it and it makes you feel good, then go for it!

I saw a woman walking down Oxford Street recently and she looked so incredible I wanted to stop her and tell her so. She must have been in her seventies and had cropped white hair, beautiful glasses, and was wearing a baggy black dress, tights and shoes, and a slash of red lipstick. She was striding along with her head up, and I could see I wasn't the only one transfixed by her awesomeness. Her age had nothing, and everything, to do with it – she was a lioness!

Look at Dame Julie Walters, too – a beautiful, funny woman whose personality twinkles out of her like fairy dust – and Dame Judi Dench, who looks as if she could swap a filthy joke or two while shining like a goddess on the red carpet. In fact, there was a wonderful story in *The Times* a while ago, involving Dame Judi, which Roger Moore recounted in his autobiography, and which I hope to God is true because it's made me love her even more. Apparently, she became distracted while crossing the road and a black cab had to swerve to avoid her. The irate driver leaned out of his window and yelled, 'Mind where you're going, you stupid ****!' To which she levelled her cool blue eyes upon him and retorted, 'It's Dame **** to you . . .' before strolling on. And if you're counting the asterisks to figure out which word she used, yes, apparently it really was *that* one!

You see? Age has nothing to do with invisibility; it's our attitude that renders us powerless or powerful. I'm not saying that a pair of trainers, wearing red lipstick or swearing back at taxi drivers is the answer for you, but I strongly believe that finding your own version of these things will go a long way to reclaiming your sense of self.

Help me, I'm knackered

I used to be the Duracell bunny and could keep going and going and going. Not now. I've always loved my sleep and as long as I got enough at some point during the week, I could handle anything. Not now. I get *so tired* I can barely stand. However, like Dory in *Finding Nemo*, I keep smiling and 'just keep swimming!' I do what I can until I can't do it any more.

It's one of the few things Nick has struggled to get his head around – how I can be full of beans for a couple of months, then will crash and not be able to move for a week, riddled with all-over body pain, anxiety, exhaustion and self-doubt. My body and brain shut down.

When I get like this I *stop*. I crawl into bed, take some Nytol and sleep and sleep. If I can. If I can't sleep, then I get a short-term prescription from my GP for some sleeping tablets, and try to break the non-sleeping cycle long enough for me to get back to normal again.

If you're feeling exhausted, don't automatically assume it's the menopause, though. Low energy levels can be the result of all sorts of other medical conditions, so it's worth talking to your GP just to make sure there's nothing else going on. If it is down to the changes the menopause brings, there's no quick-fix solution, but exercising every day (even just a small amount), drinking less caffeine and alcohol, eating a little better, learning how to relax, getting enough sleep (make sure your bedroom isn't too hot), drinking lots of water, and learning to say no to things so that you're not overly busy, will all help to restore your energy levels.

Every face tells a story

The menopause – bringing with it a decline in oestrogen levels and a reduction in collagen production – can cause your skin to change. We're getting older anyway, but the menopause can, and will, accelerate the skin's ageing process: thinning, wrinkles and sagging.

One of the things I find I'm struggling with is that my skin is so saggy! I can almost feel it dropping around my once-tight neck and I hate it. It's because all the hormonal changes cause the loss of some fat from the upper layer of your skin and a reduction in its elasticity. You might also notice the impact around your jawline and on your cheeks.

To combat wrinkles I've had Botox in my forehead. It's really to stop the severe frown I've inherited from my dad from appearing between my eyes, which causes my kids to ask constantly if I'm cross. The injections have had varying degrees of success. Sometimes I look fresh and smooth, other times I look demented – it's like a needle version of Russian roulette. Sometimes I swear I'm never going to try it again, then my face sags and I look angry when I'm not, and so I book myself in and shout 'Freeze me!' to the doctor.

I am vain and I like looking good *for my age*. I don't mind getting older. I just don't see why I should look tired and angry all the time (though, to be fair, I am!), because that's what ageing, exacerbated by the menopause, seems to do to women. It's really brutal on the skin, which is all the more reason to look after it. Here are a few ideas on how you might do that.

Moisturize. Moisturize. Moisturize.

My face has suffered from breakouts throughout different stages of my life, and hormones have always been to blame! I look after my skin, though – I always have done. Having acne in my teens meant that I've known for a long time how important it is to make sure my face is clean, moisturized and protected, and I've carried on with that regime through my adult life.

To kick off, you need to cleanse your skin with a product that won't dry it out – something creamy and hydrating. I always clean my skin with a facewash (whatever I come across in the chemist or supermarket) and a muslin cloth or flannel, and remove any eye make-up with an oil-based remover so

I don't have to rub too hard around my eyes. I then use Harley Street Skin Care Restorative Miracle Serum, Anne Semonin's Miracle Eye Contour cream (who doesn't want miracles to happen, eh?) and Liz Earle's Superskin Moisturiser every morning and night.

During and after the menopause your skin becomes drier because your oil glands aren't as active. It's more important than ever to keep your skin hydrated, so drink lots of water, but remember you might also need to invest in a heavier cream. Hydration has always been part of my skincare regime but I can't emphasize this enough: moisturize. A lot.

My little bag of make-up tricks

We've all got one. Mine is overflowing with lots of products that I own 'just in case', but there are a few essentials in there that I couldn't do without.

• IT's Bye Bye Under Eye concealer is perfect for slightly older skin that needs something to cover the problem areas but doesn't cake in the wrinkles.

• On the rest of my skin I use bareMinerals' Complexion Rescue Tinted Hydrating Gel Cream with SPF 30. It's vital to use a face product with an SPF of at least 30 every day, as your skin has less natural protection against the sun than it did when you were younger. While our bodies need vitamin D, your face won't thank you for the ageing effects of unprotected sun exposure!

• When it comes to the eyes, I have a MAC eye palette, which does pretty much everything, including eyebrows. Smashbox's X-Rated Mascara is also an essential.

- For cheeks and lips, I go for MAC's Ladyblush cream blusher, and their Patisserie lipstick.

One of the things about ageing is that you can become a bit stuck in your fashion and make-up ways. It's good to shake it up a little and try something new. Mineral make-up has come a long way over the last few years, and is a wonderful help for menopausal women, as it allows the skin to breathe. This means that when a hot flush arrives, you can sweat through it, and gently dab away any moisture without rubbing off your make-up. Lighter creams work better as well, rather than thick foundations which can become mask-like, settling into cracks and crevices!

The skin around the eyes is especially difficult to deal with, as the more make-up you put on to hide the shadows resulting from sleepless nights, the worse it can look. I prefer a serum-based concealer (Bobbi Brown have a good selection), with some light powder dusted over the top. A creamy lipstick or one of the hundreds of coloured glosses that are out there work much better than drying, matt lip liners and lipsticks.

If all else fails, I get through tins of Vaseline – I always have some in my handbag, ready to smear on to dry lips, or even hands if they feel like they need it. I also carry a cream blush with me as I can dab it on with my fingers – no need for a brush – and blend it in.

A cut above

I've never been blessed with thick hair, but before I had children I was pretty happy with it. Then, the hormones kicked in during pregnancy and my locks were luscious and full, but as their levels fell away postpartum, so too did much of my hair, and it never came back again. What I was left with was thin and crappy.

Once the menopause began, a receding hairline was added to the mix, which was bad enough, but it also coincided with a new growth of thick hair – everywhere else! The sides of my face, upper lip, and oh my God, my chin! How the hell can hair strong enough to bear the weight of a small car grow out of my chin overnight, while I can see my skull through the pathetic strands at my temples? How bloody unfair is that? Again, hormones are to blame.

The tweezers – and perhaps the lovely lady who threads and waxes at your local salon – will become your new best friend. It seems that while HRT can go a long way to alleviating many of the symptoms of the menopause, it doesn't necessarily improve the hair situation.

I can deal with growing a fuzz but I decided enough was enough with the thin hair. You can cover up your body if you're not happy with it, but losing your crowning glory is one of the toughest things to deal with as you get older – for both men and women. Long, luscious hair is such a symbol of health, vitality and, let's face it, youth. Having it ebb away, both literally and figuratively, was not something I was ready for.

As well as making your hair thin, the menopause can cause it to become dull and dry. As always, it seems, it's because you have lower levels of oestrogen and progesterone. In an attempt to improve the situation, every few weeks I use a hair oil – I work it through instead of conditioner and let it soak in. In the past, I've dabbled with hair extensions to make my hair look longer, but now I have them to thicken the damn stuff. I used to be embarrassed by this, but then I heard that Mary Berry uses them for the same reason, and she's an octogenarian cookery goddess, so it must be OK!

Extensions aren't an option for everyone, though. If you're worried about thinning hair and hair loss, you need to use really gentle products and styling techniques. Be nice to it! A good stylist will be able to help you with ways to disguise thinness, but all the things I've talked about in previous chapters – eating well (vitamin C, and protein- and iron-rich foods such as red meats, are good for hair), exercise, reducing stress and keeping hydrated – will help to keep your hair healthier and stronger during the menopause.

Long in the tooth

Skincare, hair loss, hair growth . . . All these things spring to mind immediately when you think of how your body changes during the menopause, but one of the things that you don't automatically think of is your dental health, and how your teeth and gums are affected when your hormone levels change. With the drop in oestrogen that happens during this time, your mouth is yet another part of the body that gets drier – who knew? This can lead to increased bacteria growth in your mouth, which in turn can lead to gum disease and tooth decay.

Have you ever wondered where the term 'long in the tooth' comes from? It doesn't just mean 'old', it means you're showing more of your teeth because your gums are receding – another thing associated with old age. Receding gums also mean your teeth can start moving about, and in my case, they became more crooked than ever, especially at the bottom.

Those of you who watch *Loose Women* regularly may

remember a time early in 2016 when I looked like my mouth had exploded. I received many comments about it on social media, and most of them were saying things such as, 'WTF has Andrea McLean done to her lips?' The answer was . . . nothing. I hadn't done anything to my lips, but I *had* done something to my teeth. I'd decided to have braces. Full-on, metal-mouth, in-yer-face braces. To try to hold back the years, I was now holding back the tears – they hurt! I decided to do it then because my son, Fin, had just had his fitted. I was supposed to have braces as a teen, but had chickened out, and as I saw him lying bravely in the dentist's chair, I thought, 'What kind of mum am I, to tell him how brave he's being, when I couldn't do it myself?' So the time seemed right, and I thought it could be something we could go through together.

The theory behind getting braces in middle age was a good one: they would pull my ivories back into place and put a halt to the tombstone-tooth effect I had going on. In practice, things weren't so simple. The metal version affected the way I spoke and looked; I was lisping and spitting on air, and looked as if I'd had a very bad lip job. After just a month I swapped to Invisalign – which are removable and a great alternative to traditional orthodontic braces, not least because they're virtually invisible. They suited me much better, as I could take them out before I went on TV, so that I looked and sounded the same. Then I'd pop them back in as soon I was finished. I wore them for just under two years, but I'm so glad I had them, as I now have the smile I've always wanted. My teeth are strong and held in place by a small wire bonded to the back of my teeth so they won't go on a menopausal walkabout any more.

Going for major dental treatment in your forties might seem like an extravagance, but it's a fact that your gums and teeth *will* change as your hormones affect your body. Whether you do it because you don't like how they look, or because you want to safeguard them for the future, I'd definitely recommend doing all you can to look after your teeth before they become a real problem.

In the old days, damaged teeth used to be pulled out and falsies were dished out like, well, sweeties. Both my grannies had a full mouth of false teeth by the time they were my age. Nowadays, as long as we look after our teeth and gums, the only falsies on our face should be lashes!

There are various quick wins that don't involve some serious shelling out. Invest in an electric toothbrush, if you don't already have one. Brush for two minutes after every meal but also start flossing and rinsing with mouthwash, all of which will help to combat gum disease. Also think about getting your teeth professionally cleaned more often – at least every six months. You're aiming to minimize the number of places where food particles can get stuck and form plaque, which is at the heart of tooth decay. If you find yourself grinding your teeth – an increasingly common way for stress to manifest itself – make sure to invest in a night guard.

Tell your face!

Can I be honest here? I've been searingly honest about myself, but now I'm going to be honest about *you* . . . This is an observation and you're probably not going to like it, but see it for what it is – a gentle nudge from a friend who cares about you. Never mind make-up and skincare routines, SPF chat, antioxidants and yoga routines, just watch your resting bitch face. I see so many women looking thoroughly pissed off, at anything and everything, and if there's a sure-fire way of making yourself look older, it's by walking around with a face like a bulldog chewing a wasp.

I get it. I have days like that, where *everyone and everything* gets on my nerves. Sure, sometimes it's them (you're right, some people are excruciatingly annoying) but a lot of the time, it's *you*. During the menopause your annoyance radar is up and swivelling, and *anything* will drive you mad. Try to remember that and either accept it, or make allowances for it. And if you're in a good mood, *tell your face*. It'll knock years off you.

How do you know when it's over?

I had my hysterectomy at the end of 2016, and a year and a half later I'm still swinging from emotional rope to emotional rope like a hormonal Jane of the Jungle. I have good days and bad days. I still suffer from crippling, all-encompassing anxiety where my whole body hurts, from my skin to my hair. I break out in mouth ulcers, I feel exhausted and run-down, and at night my heart beats so hard and my stomach churns so much that I can't for the life of me fall asleep. When I do, I wake in the small hours, agonizing over everything that could go wrong in my life, catastrophizing until I'm a ball of teeth-clenching, head-aching stress.

One night I lay awake worrying that Donald Trump would cause World War Three, which would lead to Armageddon and – get this – there would be no more HRT in the world, and what would I do then? Never mind the fact that we could all be wiped out, or turned into zombies, or whatever; the burning issue was what the hell would happen to me if I couldn't get my hormones!

After days, possibly weeks, of terrible nights I can wake up one day and not feel so bad. The fear has ebbed away like a toxic wave. These are just my personal fears – we all have our own anxieties that keep us awake at night, swivel-eyed with worry that our imagination-spun fictions will become fact. I've decided that from now on I'm going to start writing my fears down as part of my penchant for journalling.

Rather than lying there in the dark, becoming more and more agitated and stressed about something that probably isn't going to happen (I really hope so in the case of zombies), if it's written down then a) it's out of your head and your mind will let go of its tight, hysterical grip on it, and b) when you read it in the morning you will realize just how ridiculous you were being, which will hopefully stop you worrying about it again. It's worth a go.

Do you ever get over the menopause? Is there a time when it's over? To be perfectly honest, I don't think there's a yes or no answer to this, because it depends on what the word 'over' means to you. Will you feel as you did before it started, like you did in your twenties and thirties? Of course not. But will you feel better than you did when your body was going through one of its biggest life changes? Probably.

Many women report feeling a huge sense of well-being once they're postmenopausal, and a contentment about who and where they are at this stage in their life. Some have more energy and confidence because they've found what works for them, to make them feel good. I think that if we use this time to really look deeply within ourselves, to find what works for us as individuals in terms of how we look after our bodies and minds, then once we reach the other side, we're in a better position to live a healthy, happy life, which is all any of us can hope for.

The bright side

If I can end on one last piece of advice, it has to be the philosophy I try my best to live by, even when I'm anxious and stressed, or feeling awful in some way because of what life is throwing at me: 'It is what it is . . .'

I try to make the most of what I have right now, rather than thinking about what I don't have, or how things should or could be. It really does help to look on the positive side of things, even when it doesn't feel as if there is one. There are a lot of things out there to make you feel bad, either about yourself or about life in general, and only we can choose how to react to them. Self-pity is the killer of joy, and it's joy that puts a spring in your step and a twinkle in your eye. Feel the joy, keep the twinkle – that's what will see you through.

Look around you: there are so many *incredible* women of a certain age doing fabulously well by completely being themselves, accepting who they are and not wishing they were younger, faster, prettier, fresher . . . We are *amazing*! If you've hit a pothole on your journey, recognize it for what it is and drive on. Your teeth may be clenched, you may be convinced one of your tyres is going to fall off and your suspension is broken, but it's probably not that bad . . . Things may not be in perfect working order, but it's usually possible to navigate your way down the road none the less.

And if something really is broken, we can try our best to fix it. There are so many things that you can do to help yourself. Most of all, we can help one another by talking to one another. That's what friends are for.

Dr Peers Says . . .

FIGHTING FATIGUE

Fatigue is a common problem during the menopause. Hormone imbalance, lifestyle stressors and menopause symptoms that affect your sleep, such as night sweats and insomnia, can lead to tiredness. Sadly, it can increase stress and anxiety levels, which in turn causes insomnia and makes things worse. The good news is that there are things you can do to help:

• Make sure you have a good sleep routine – go to bed and wake at the same time each day, avoid stimulants such as caffeine and alcohol at bedtime, and switch off screens at least an hour before going to bed.

• Keep your bedroom well ventilated to reduce night sweats.

• Exercise regularly; even if it's only walking for 15 to 20 minutes each day, it can help with energy levels.

• Try relaxation exercises and meditation, or try yoga or tai chi to reduce stress.

• Take a short nap – even 10 minutes can help to relieve fatigue.

• Use aromatherapy oils, such as lavender, sandalwood or jasmine, on your pillow or by your bed at night to help you sleep.[1]

SKIN AND HAIR WOES – THE SCIENCE . . .

Declining oestrogen levels can affect your skin in many ways. Reduced blood flow to the skin means that it doesn't receive the same levels of nutrients and oxygen as it did before the menopause. As a result, the cell-renewal process is reduced, water loss is increased and skin can become dry. Loss of natural oils resulting from lower oestrogen levels also plays a part in drying out the skin.

Oestrogen also helps with the production of collagen, an important component for healthy skin and prevention of premature ageing. As a result, the skin becomes less elastic and more prone to sagging and wrinkles. In women on HRT, the oestrogen receptors in the fibroblasts in the skin respond to the oestrogen in HRT, resulting in an increase in the production of collagen. Many women notice an improvement in their skin, hair and nails after commencing HRT. Collagen is also in our muscles, joints and intervertebral discs. It cushions the joints and protects them from damage when we exercise.

Loss of melanin at this time can also make your skin more prone to sun damage. There are apps available that help you monitor your exposure to summer sun and recommend the appropriate SPFs to minimize damage.

As women age, the pattern and speed of hair growth can change. During the menopause, it may mean that you notice thinning hair at the crown or around the hairline – a condition known as female pattern hair loss (FPHL). It's very common and influenced by both hormones and genetics, so there well may be a family link. Losing your hair is upsetting but a healthy balanced diet can help to slow the loss and, in severe cases, cosmetic and medical treatments are available to help improve long-term hair growth.

1 *Source: Menopause Health Matters. Menopause Insomnia. www.menopausehealthmatters.com*

2 *Sources: Menopause Health Matters. Menopause Insomnia. www.menopausehealthmatters.com; Women's Health Concern. Menopausal Skin Changes. www.womens-health-concern.org*

Appendix

In a Nutshell

As a Consultant in Contraception and Reproductive Health, with a particular interest in the management of the meno-pause, Dr Tina Peers has, as she puts it, the 'great privilege and joy' of being able to help many women as they experi-ence the perimenopause and then become postmenopausal. Here's her final word and bottom line on what you need to know about the menopause.

Menopausal symptoms

The menopause refers to a woman's last menstrual period. I think it's actually more helpful to refer to this time as the climacteric, as this is the period of time – up to ten years or more – over which a woman's hormones and ovarian function gradually diminish and result in the presence of around thirty-four physical symptoms (see page 10).

On a daily basis, I see women struggling with symptoms, which are caused by the fluctuating levels of hormones dur-ing the climacteric or by being postmenopausal. As many of these symptoms creep into their lives, women put them down to tiredness, stress, or simply see them as part of be-coming middle-aged. Cruelly, this all happens at a time in a woman's life when she's often trying to be all things to all people! She may still have children to look after (their demands can still be considerable, even when they're older), a partner, a household to run, a career and, more often than not in this day and age, elderly parents to care for.

It may also be a time in a woman's life when she's only just getting into her stride, with new-found freedoms from looking after a young family, possibly a little more disposable income for travel and leisure, and her career might be taking off. She needs and wants to feel fit, well and full of energy, not debilitated by hot flushes, poor-quality sleep, anxiety and sometimes depression. These menopausal symptoms can certainly impact negatively on a woman's quality of life!

Things aren't helped by a loss of libido, vaginal dryness, and discomfort during intercourse. No matter how loving a woman's relationship with her partner may be, we know that an active sex life enhances that relationship and feeling of intimacy.

A survey was conducted by my friend Professor Rossella Nappi in Pavia, into attitudes surrounding sex and the effect sex has on a relationship. She says, as a result of her research, that good sex contributes about 30 per cent to the happiness in a relationship, but an absence of it takes away about 70 per cent. I think this is because men and women are fundamentally quite different when it comes to sex. Women need affection to feel like having sex with their partner; men need sex to give affection. If sex happens less frequently, men stop being affectionate and so there'll be even less sex! I know this is a generalization, but it's backed by research and many women I see confirm that it tallies with their experience.

Contraception and fertility in the climacteric

I also see women for their contraception needs as they approach the menopause – a time when they're potentially still fertile and therefore need, or want, to prevent pregnancy. Contraception should continue to be used for two years if a woman's last menstrual period occurs before the age of fifty, and for one year if it occurs after that age.

Of course, some forms of hormonal contraception can mask the signs of the menopause, and make it difficult to know when it has happened. Progestogen-only methods may stop monthly bleeds completely. For example, many women choose to use the very safe and convenient intrauterine hormonal device for their contraception. Its local action in the womb usually stops heavy periods and bleeding altogether, and can be extremely helpful at this time in a woman's life when periods often become heavier, longer and more frequent.

Understandably, these women ask me how they'll know when their periods have stopped and they're actually post-menopausal. The hormonal intrauterine device contains a progestogen hormone, I tell them, but no oestrogen. Therefore, any signs of oestrogen deficiency that occur at the menopause won't be masked and will give women using such a device a strong indication that they've become menopausal. These women will also be in the very happy position of being able to use transdermal oestrogen (a patch or daily gel) so that their symptoms are controlled and subside.

Doctors generally don't perform blood tests to confirm

the menopause if a woman is over the age of forty-five and experiencing menopausal symptoms. We base our diagnosis on the clinical picture alone. If, however, a woman is under the age of forty-five, then blood tests are recommended as it's important not to miss a diagnosis of premature menopause (menopause before the age of forty-five) and premature ovarian insufficiency (menopause before the age of forty).

Premature ovarian insufficiency (POI)

This is the loss of ovarian activity before a woman reaches the age of forty and, of course, it can be a devastating diagnosis. Spontaneous POI affects 1 to 6 per cent of women below that age; however, increasing numbers of women are affected as a result of cancer treatments or surgery. The causes are mostly unknown, genetic or connected to auto-immune diseases. Women who have POI experience the symptoms of the climacteric and also find themselves at increased risk of cardiovascular disease, osteoporosis and premature cognitive decline. Their life expectancy can be reduced if POI is undiagnosed and untreated. The diagnosis also obviously has implications for a woman's fertility.

Premature ovarian insufficiency has important differences from the 'normal' menopause, which occurs at the average age of fifty-one in the UK. The average age at which POI is diagnosed is, surprisingly, thirty-one years old. It's essential that a woman with POI receives specialist help and advice to restore her hormone balance, protect her bones, cardiovascular system, cognitive function, muscles, bladder and vaginal health, libido and feeling of well-being with HRT. This therapy should be taken until the age of fifty-two at least, and many women will choose to continue on their HRT into their sixties and seventies, and beyond.

The ovarian production of hormones and eggs can fluctuate in POI (the ovaries have not failed irreversibly) and result in the occasional period and even pregnancy. About 5–10 per cent of women with POI will conceive naturally. Therefore, if pregnancy is not desired, contraception must be considered.

Women of this age who have not yet had a family but would like one should be referred to an Assisted Conception Unit. I'd recommend that any woman who has experienced four months of menstrual irregularities should consult her GP, no matter how young she is, as we need to consider and exclude this diagnosis. Missing POI can be very detrimental to a woman's health.

For more information on POI, please contact the charity the Daisy Network, an excellent resource which has a very useful website and provides valuable support and information for women with POI: www.daisynetwork.org.uk.

The idea of a 'fertility holiday'

When women are using the combined contraceptive pill, they may do so for many years. During this time, ovulation is inhibited and bleeds are induced in the hormone-free interval of each cycle. Some mini-pills also prevent ovulation, and both types of contraception could well be masking the signs of POI. It's therefore a good idea for women to consider having a 'fertility holiday' in their late twenties to mid-thirties to check their ovarian reserve.

This means stopping taking the pill, and using another method of contraception for two to three months, in order to check their fertility status. Blood tests and ultrasound scans can determine whether the pill has been concealing any underlying fertility problems. Not all methods of contraception are anovulatory (prevent ovulation). Intrauterine devices, for example, both copper and hormonal devices, act locally and don't inhibit a woman's natural cycle and so the appropriate tests can be carried out without having to stop using these methods.

I'd recommend that all women consider an ovarian reserve test by the age of thirty – and by the age of thirty-five at the latest, when a woman's fertility starts to decline naturally.

Accessing the right information

Once a woman has done some research and reading on the subject of the menopause, I'd recommend an appointment with a GP, some of whom are well informed and experienced in menopause management. However, women who have more complex medical histories, or feel that they would like further assistance, should, in my opinion, consult someone with a special interest in and experience of menopause management. HRT can then be discussed with whichever medical professional they decide to see, the potential risks and benefits will be explained fully, and a personal regimen tailored to the woman's needs, response and stage of her menopausal journey can be devised. With HRT, it's not a case of 'one size fits all' – the therapy needs monitoring and careful adjustment.

The symptoms that women may experience during the menopause can come on gradually – or indeed quite suddenly – and last, on average, for ten to twelve years. During this time, these symptoms can be alleviated by taking HRT or using various non-hormonal complementary alternative remedies. Non-hormonal remedies that can be bought over the counter should be used with caution, and I'd only recommend those with clinical data to show that they actually improve the symptoms, such as red clover (80mg a day) and Femal, a new food supplement that will soon be available in the UK, made from the cytoplasm of pollen (one tablet a day).

The websites below contain a comprehensive list of alternative therapies to help menopausal women and further information about their potential risks and benefits. (NB The use of red clover, black cohosh, vitamin E and magnetic devices is *not* recommended by NICE (the National Institute for Health and Care Excellence) for the management of menopause symptoms in women with breast cancer.)

When discussing and prescribing HRT, every woman needs to have an individual assessment that considers her family history, her medical history and her personal preferences. Generally, specialists favour 'body-identical', pharmaceutically made, regulated HRT preparations that are identical to the natural hormones produced by the woman's own body. They are manufactured from yams, and clinical data and studies show that they are safe and effective to use. This is always a good place to start.

There are many myths about the risks of HRT and it's difficult for women to source accurate information that can help them make an informed decision about using HRT. I'd recommend the NICE Guidelines on Menopause Management information for women, published in November 2015: www.nice.org.uk/guidance/ng23/ifp/chapter/About-this-information; the British Menopause Society website: www.womens-health-concern.org/help-and-advice/factsheets/menopause/; and the website of my colleague Dr Heather Currie: www.menopausematters.co.uk.

Proven benefits of HRT

Not only does HRT help to improve the quality of women's lives while they are in the climacteric – which can last for ten to twelve years, remember – but it also provides positive long-term benefits when it comes to future health and well-being.

• A meta-analysis of randomized controlled trials from 1966 to September 2002 of 26,708 women with an average age of fifty-four showed a significant reduction in mortality (39 per cent) in women less than sixty years of age.[1]
• HRT helps maintain bone density and these benefits are maintained many years after stopping HRT.[2] One of my patients, aged sixty-three, first discovered that she had

osteoporosis when her husband picked her up to demonstrate his strength to his grandchildren. He broke three of her ribs by just lifting her.

• HRT benefits the cardiovascular system. In women aged fifty to fifty-nine, there is no increased risk of coronary heart disease or stroke, with a 30 per cent reduction in any cause of mortality.[3]

• HRT reduces the risk of colorectal cancer by 30 per cent.[4]

• HRT has also been shown to reduce the incidence of cognitive decline.[5]

Potential risks of HRT

As with any medication, the benefits of taking it have to be balanced with the risks.

• In a woman with no uterus, there is no apparent excess risk for breast cancer after five years of HRT use. In fact, in the WHI study there was a statistically significant reduced risk. However, there may be a very small increased risk of breast cancer with some types of HRT. We have data to show that this small increase (possibly one extra case per 1,200 women per year on HRT) then reverts back to the normal risk five years after stopping the HRT.

Each woman needs to be counselled on an individual basis, and the advice will vary depending on her family history and her own medical history. However, it should be remembered that the risk of breast cancer is increased significantly by other factors, such as obesity and alcohol consumption. It's therefore important to keep the risk of HRT balanced with the potential benefits.

• The risk of blood clots is not increased if oestrogen is administered transdermally (through the skin). Oral oestrogen increases the blood-clotting factors minimally and temporarily. Again, other factors that increase this risk in women, such as obesity and smoking, should be considered when thinking about the risks of taking HRT.

• There is no increased risk of endometrial cancer in continuous combined HRT.

Hysterectomies and HRT

Women who have had a hysterectomy, unless for endometriosis, can have oestrogen-only HRT. We have data to show that this actually reduces their risk of breast cancer by 27 per cent.[6]

Oestrogen can be taken in the form of a gel, patch, tablet or implant. Oestrogen gels and patches are preferable as they don't increase the production of clotting factors (something that oral oestrogen does temporarily for a few weeks after starting the therapy), do not affect cholesterol adversely, and may indeed reduce the bad cholesterol.

Progestogens need to be taken as part of their HRT by women who still have their uterus, or who have had a hysterectomy for endometriosis. This is to protect the endometrial tissue and prevent it becoming thickened under the influence of the oestrogen. Progestogens can come in the form of patches or tablets, or be delivered via the intrauterine five-year device that is also licensed for contraception. Natural, micronized progesterone is generally well tolerated and often helps women sleep better – an absolute blessing!

Some women may also be prescribed a drug known as a SERM – Selective Estrogen Receptor Modulator – which has been designed to maximize the benefits of HRT and minimize the side effects. These modulators act in different ways, depending on which hormone receptor they bind to and switch on or off, and not all are licensed for HRT use. Two new SERM preparations are licensed in the UK for use in the menopause – Ospemifene, for the treatment of vaginal atrophy, and Duavive, a combination therapy which can be useful in some women who are progestogen intolerant but want to benefit from HRT. Ospemifene can be used to treat vaginal atrophy in women who have had breast cancer in the past, once they have completed their treatment for the cancer.

A note on testosterone

This is a really important hormone for both men and women. It may come as a surprise but women actually have four times as many testosterone receptors as oestrogen receptors. Testosterone is produced by the ovaries and adrenals, and the latter continue to produce it after the menopause.

Testosterone deficiency symptoms include low libido, tearfulness, low mood, lack of energy, poor concentration, weaker or absent orgasms, and a general loss of *joie de vivre*. Many women really enjoy the benefits of testosterone gel when prescribed to help with these symptoms. It often helps to restore their 'get-up-and-go', can benefit their bones and heart, and may also help with weight loss.

So how long can I stay on HRT?

The NICE Guidelines for Menopause Management categorically state that 'there is no arbitrary cut-off to the length of time a woman can take HRT, it is purely up to the individual. She should be supported in her decision to continue it if she desires this.'

Once they experience the feeling of wellness, the return of their energy and vitality, the increase in their libido, the improvement in the quality of their lives on HRT, many, *many* of my patients are loath to stop taking it after five, ten, fifteen, twenty years. There is actually no time limit on how long you can take HRT for.

One of the most satisfying parts of my job is helping women to feel well again, get their bounce back and help them to understand how to keep well into their old age. 'Thank you for giving me my life back,' is music to my ears!

1 *Salpeter, S.R., Walsh, J.M., Greyber, E., et al. 'Mortality associated with hormone replacement therapy in younger and older women: a meta-analysis'. J Gen Intern Med 2004; 19(7): 791–804.*

2 *Huang, A., Grady, D., Blackwell, T., Bauer, D. 'Hot flushes, bone mineral density, and fractures in older postmenopausal women'. Obstet Gynecol 2007; 109(4): 841–7.*

Appendix

3 La Croix, A.Z., Chlebowski, R.T., Manson, J.E., et al; WHI Investigators. 'Health outcomes after stopping conjugated equine estrogens among postmenopausal women with prior hysterectomy: a randomized controlled trial'. JAMA 2011; 305(13): 1305–14.

4 Manson, J.E., Chlebowski, R.T., Stefanick, M.L., et al. 'Menopausal hormone therapy and health outcomes during the intervention and extended poststopping phases of the Women's Health Initiative randomized trials'. JAMA 2013; 310(13): 1353–68.

Harz, A., He, T., Rimm, A. Comparison of adiposity measures as risk factors in postmenopausal women. J Clin Endocrinol Metab 2012; 97(1): 227–33.

5 Carlson, M. C. et al. Hormone replacement therapy and reduced cognitive decline in older women: the Cache County Study. Neurology 2001: 57(12): 2210–16.

6 Women's Health Initiative Steering Committee. 'Effects of conjugated equine estrogens in postmenopausal women with hysterectomy.' The Women's Health Initiative Randomized Controlled Trial. JAMA 2004; 291: 1701–12.

Acknowledgements

I couldn't have written this book without the help and support of many people. Literally, thousands of people! First of all, thank you to all of you who contacted me after my first wobbly announcement on TV that I was going to be having a hysterectomy; expressing concern, asking me questions, and sharing your experiences. This book wouldn't have been written if you hadn't let me know how desperate you are to talk about this fundamental part of a woman's life. Thank you to all the wonderful and honest women who answered my questions on Facebook and Twitter, joined me during my live discussions, and passed on your stories. I hope I've done you proud.

Thank you to Linda Robson for outing me on the telly. You do realize you started something with your baggy mouth, don't you? Thank you to *all* my lovely Loose Women – the ones on TV and the ones behind the scenes – for being such great friends. You're amazing.

Thank you to Dr Tina Peers, MBBS, DRCOG, DFSRH, FFSRH, MBCAM, Consultant in Contraception and Reproductive Health, and to Lynn Hamilton, BSc, MA, Medical Writer and Editor, who have provided the invaluable medical information and advice which is peppered throughout this book, and ensures that you really are armed with everything you need to know about the menopause.

Thank you to my agent, Jonny McWilliams, for not running for the hills when I said I wanted to write a book for menopausal women that allowed them to ask questions and to have their say. You may not have jumped *fully* on board when I pestered you into getting behind this, but it's been brilliant watching your understanding of what a huge subject this is, to the point where even *you* are now badgering others to get involved! Thank you for putting up with my calls, emails, to-do lists, goals, aims, hopes and dreams, and for helping me to make them a reality. There will be a *new* list of goals, aims, hopes and dreams pinging into your inbox now this is done, Jonny, so brace yourself.

Thank you to my literary agent, Carly Cook, who from our very first meeting calmly took in my overzealous, arm-waving enthusiasm about the importance of a book that let menopausal women roar, and agreed with me. This book wouldn't have come to light if it weren't for you. I think you're amazing, and I hope this is the start of many books to come. *Menopausal Maldives*, perhaps? I think that has a ring to it . . .

Thank you to Andrea Henry and the fantastic team at Transworld for believing in this book and editing my words so that they flow and make sense. It has been a joy working with you all.

Thank you to copy editor Rebecca Wright for brilliantly pointing out the bits that didn't make sense (I do love to mix my metaphors) and coaxing much more out of me when I thought I'd said it all.

Thank you to my brother-in-law John Feeney for going through my recipes and giving them a little extra boost. It's very handy having a master chef in the family!

To my lovely family – Mum, Dad and Linda – for your enthusiasm and support. Just knowing you've got my back makes me less frightened of falling. And Mum, thank you for allowing me to use your special soup recipe – who knows, it could get passed down through other families now?

Thank you, Lin, for looking after me. I think we both know I need you much more than the kids do – you're my right-hand woman, my sounding board, and my 'other mum'.

Thank you, kids – Finlay, Amy, Tia Lily and Sienna – for bearing with me while I sat hunched over my computer in the office, and for understanding that I wasn't always able to join in with stuff. 'I'm writing . . .' has been a bit of a catchphrase in our house lately, and you'll be pleased to know you've got me back again!

Last, but not least, thank you to my husband, Nick. Thank you for letting me talk about us in this book, even the embarrassing stuff. Thank you for bearing with me while I raged, understanding when I've slid into darkness, coaxing me out of myself when I've anxiously hidden from the world, supporting me when I've stepped into the light, and believing in me at every stage. You came into my life when I least expected it, and have helped me through some of the most difficult experiences of my life – and that's saying something! You make me laugh, you listen to me, and you were the only person to point out that bootcut jeans really don't suit me – for that alone I will always be grateful. I love you to the moon and back.

Andrea McLean is one of the primary anchors on the award-winning ITV lunchtime talk show *Loose Women*. Before she joined the show in 2007, she was best known as one of the core team of presenters on the ITV breakfast programme *GMTV*. Andrea has just celebrated her twenty-first year with ITV. She began her career as a freelance travel writer and has gone on to write for *Red, Best, Scottish Woman*, the *Mirror* and numerous women's weekly magazines. Her autobiography, *Confessions of a Good Girl*, was a *Sunday Times* number one bestseller.